Core Concepts in Pharmacology

Manuchair Ebadi, Ph.D.

Professor of Pharmacology, Neurology, and Psychiatry
University of Nebraska College of Medicine, Omaha

Illustrations by Mike Chance

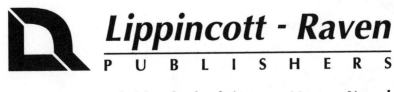

Lippincott - Raven
P U B L I S H E R S

Philadelphia • New York

Copyright © 1997 by Lippincott-Raven Publishers

First Edition

Library of Congress Cataloging-in-Publication Data

Ebadi, Manuchair S.
    Core concepts in pharmacology / Manuchair Ebadi ; illustrations by
Mike Chance.
       p.   cm.
    Includes index.
    ISBN 0-316-19952-4 (pbk.)
    1. Pharmacology.   I. Title.
    [DNLM: 1. Pharmacology.   2. Drug Therapy.   QV 4 E15c   1997]
RM300.E328   1997
615′.1 — dc20
DNLM/DLC
for Library of Congress   96-27696
                                            CIP

Printed in the United States of America

VICTOR GRAPHICS, INC.

Production Services: Textbook Writers Associates, Inc.

Copyeditor: Beverly Miller

Indexer: Michael Loo

Designer: Linda Dana Willis

Cover Design: Hannus Design Associates

This book is humbly and reverently dedicated to patients everywhere,
who yearn to be relieved from their physical and mental suffering,
and to physicians everywhere, who, as an extension of the Lord
Almighty, are able to care and bring peace to their patients.

In books lies the soul of the whole past time, the articulate audible voice of the past when the body and material substance of it has altogether vanished like a dream.

Thomas Carlyle

Contents

Preface   ix

Introduction   xi

I. Principles of Pharmacology

1. The Pharmacokinetic Basis of Therapeutics   3

2. Pharmacodynamics   10

3. Adverse Reactions and Drug-Drug Interactions   12

II. Autonomic Pharmacology

4. The Autonomic Nervous System   17

III. Neuropharmacology

5. Drugs for Parkinson's Disease   31

6. Anticonvulsants   37

IV. Psychopharmacology

7. The Neuroleptics and Schizophrenia   47

8. Anxiolytic Agents   53

9. Antidepressants   56

V. Central Nervous System Pharmacology

10. Narcotic Analgesics   67

11. Analgesics-Antipyretics and Antiinflammatory Agents   71

12. General, Spinal, and Local Anesthetics   74

13. Skeletal Muscle Relaxants   78

14. Sedatives, Hypnotics, and Alcohol   83

VI. Diuretics and Cardiovascular Pharmacology

15. Cardiac Glycosides and Congestive Heart Failure   89

16. Antiarrhythmic Drugs   92

17. Diuretics   95

18. Vasodilators, Hypotensives, and Antihypertensive Medications   98

19. Antianginal Drugs   101

20. Anticoagulants and Thrombolytic Agents   103

21. Hematinics   106

22. Treatment of Hyperlipoproteinemias   108

VII. Endocrine Pharmacology

23. Antidiabetic Agents   111

24. Adrenal Steroids   116

25. Thyroid Hormones and Their Antagonists   122

26. Vitamin D, Calcium Homeostasis, Parathyroid Hormone, and Calcitonin   126

27. Hypothalamic and Pituitary Hormones   129

28. Reproductive Pharmacology   131

VIII. Gastrointestinal and Pulmonary Pharmacology

29. Gastrointestinal Pharmacology   137

30. Pulmonary Pharmacology   141

IX. Pharmacology of Signal Transduction and the Second-Messenger System

31. Autacoids   147

32. Eicosanoids   149

33. Hormones and Neurotransmitters Activating the Cellular Signal Transduction System   151

34. Calcium and Calcium Channel Blocking Agents **153**

X. Antimicrobial Chemotherapy and Therapy of Tuberculosis and Parasitic Diseases

35. Antimicrobial Chemotherapy **157**

36. Antifungal Agents **165**

37. Therapy of Helminthic, Protozoal, and Mycobacterial Diseases **166**

XI. Antiviral Agents, Immunopharmacology, and Cancer Chemotherapy

38. Antiviral Agents **171**

39. Immunopharmacology and Cancer Chemotherapy **173**

XII. Poisons and Antidotes

40. Treatment of Poisoning **183**

Index **187**

Preface

Hippocrates (460–377 B.C.) lamented that "life is short, and the art long; the occasion fleeting; experience fallacious; and judgment difficult." My purpose in preparing *Core Concepts in Pharmacology* was to summarize and simplify important and fundamental knowledge of pharmacology and therapeutics in an interesting and memorable fashion, and to assist students of medicine in preparing themselves for their various examinations effectively and efficiently.

I extend my respectful accolades and gratitude to Evan R. Schnittman, brilliant medical editor, formerly of Little, Brown and Company, for creating the Core Concept Series and for extending an invitation to write a book for the series. Mr. Schnittman, who has an excellent and visionary comprehension of medical education, is able to provide his authors with meaningful and insightful direction and guidance without stifling their innovative activities or creative flow.

I extend my heartfelt appreciation to Suzanne Jeans, editorial assistant, for her organizational skills, administrative support, and incomparable efficiency and attention to detail, which facilitated the completion of this book.

I gratefully acknowledge the support of Anne Holm, production editor at Little, Brown. I am thankful for the skillful input and dedication of Betty Barrer, project manager at Textbook Writers Associates, Inc., and the other professionals at TWA, Michael Loo, Beverly Miller, Melissa Ray, Rose Sklare, and Marty Tenney.

I remain eternally indebted and grateful to Mike Chance for designing, developing, and drawing the illustrations in a vivid and magnificent fashion.

I have been blessed with endearing friendship and the excellent secretarial skills of Margaret McCall, Dorothy Panowicz, Lori Clapper, Connie Curro, and Mary Overton in preparing this book.

I have always been guided by two time-honored and golden nuggets in educating my students:

> The purpose of education is to teach the young to educate themselves throughout their lives.

> Knowledge is the accumulation of science; and wisdom lies in its simplification.

I hope that this book will become a valuable tool for students in their quest for knowledge of pharmacology and therapeutics and in mastering the art of medicine.

M. E.

Introduction

Appropriate drug therapy can improve the quality of life, whereas injudicious drug therapy may result in drug-induced diseases. Physicians and dentists administer medications for diagnostic, prophylactic, or therapeutic purposes. The prescribed medications bring about the desired effects in most patients but may also prove to be inert and ineffective in some or may result in totally unexpected responses and precipitate serious reactions in others.

Iatrogenic diseases and medication-induced problems could possibly be reduced substantially if physicians or other members of the health care delivery team were fully acquainted with the principles of pharmacokinetics and remained constantly cognizant of possible unexpected interactions between drugs and ailing human bodies. One way to avoid overdosage and at the same time enhance the efficacy and safety of drug therapy is to prescribe drugs according to the achieved plasma concentrations of drugs in their active forms, not according to body weight. This practice is often essential in patients in whom the rate of absorption, distribution, biotransformation, and excretion of drugs is developing, is declining, or is altered, such as in pediatric and geriatric patients and patients with genetic abnormalities. Similarly, this practice is useful in chronically medicated individuals, such as patients with epilepsy, Parkinson's disease, or endocrine or metabolic disorders, in whom the treatment may have to be continued throughout their lifetime.

Pharmacology can be defined as the study of the selective biologic activity of chemical substances in living matter. Often, but not always, these selective biologic activities are triggered by very small amounts of drugs. For example, in treating hypothyroidism, one gives a daily dose of 50 µg of thyroxine for 1 to 2 weeks, a daily dose of 100 µg for 3 to 4 weeks, and then a permanent daily dose of approximately 150 µg. Similarly, the recommended daily allowance of vitamin B_{12} is small, being 0.5 µg in infants and 3.0 µg in adults. Dactinomycin is used in doses of 15 µg/kg/day for 5 days in the treatment of hospitalized patients with Wilms' tumor.

The effects of a drug should be selective, and the responses should occur in some but not all of the cells. Acetylcholine, which produces widespread cholinergic actions with a short duration of action, is not useful as a drug. Methacholine, carbachol, and bethanechol, the synthetic derivatives of acetylcholine, are resistant to hydrolysis and are more specific in their actions. The recognition of adrenergic receptor subtypes as $alpha_1$, $alpha_2$, $beta_1$, and $beta_2$ has resulted in the synthesis of highly specific agonists and antagonists for adrenergic receptor sites. For example, stimulation of $beta_1$ receptors causes cardiac stimulation and lipolysis, whereas stimulation of $beta_2$ is responsible for bronchodilation and vasodepression. $Beta_2$ agonists are especially useful in the treatment of asthma because they produce bronchodilation without much cardiac acceleration.

The use of drugs in the treatment of a disease is termed pharmacotherapeutics. In managing a disease, however, it is not always necessary to use drugs. **A drug may be used substitutively, supportively, prophylactically, symptomatically, diagnostically, or correctively.** For example, in type I (insulin-dependent) diabetes mellitus and Addison's disease, insulin and cortisone acetate are used, respectively, as substitutes for substances that either were never produced or were at one time but are not now produced. In type II (non-insulin-dependent) diabetes mellitus, oral hypoglycemic agents support the physiologic function of the body by stimulating the release of insulin. Although in some feverish individuals an antipyretic such as acetylsalicylic acid (aspirin) is used to reduce fever, there are infections, such as neurosyphilis, some gonococcal infections, and chronic brucellosis, in which pyrexia seems to be beneficial to the host.

Oral contraceptive tablets are used to prevent pregnancy. Isoniazid may be used to prevent the development of active tuberculosis in those individuals who have been exposed to the disease but show no evidence of infection, in those who test positively for it but have no apparent disease, and in those with active disease.

Drugs may eliminate or reduce the symptoms of a disease without influencing the actual pathology. For example, fever may be associated with respiratory tract infection, bacterial endocarditis, biliary tract disorders, tuberculosis, carcinoma, cirrhosis of the liver, collagen disease, leukemia, measles, mumps, and plague, to name a few. Aspirin can reduce the fever in these disorders but cannot alter the disease processes themselves.

A drug may also be used to diagnose a disease. Histamine has been used to assess the ability of the stomach to secrete acid and to determine parietal cell mass. If anacidity or hyposecretion occurs in response to histamine administration, this may indicate pernicious anemia, atrophic gastritis, or gastric carcinoma; a hypersecretory response may be observed in patients with duodenal ulcer or Zollinger-Ellison syndrome.

In most cases, drugs do not cure diseases, but do ease or eliminate the associated symptoms. For example, antidiarrheal agents check diarrhea, and laxatives correct constipation. No drugs exist that cure essential hypertension, but there are some that lower blood pressure. No drugs have been synthesized that cure arthritis, although a number of them reduce the pain and immobility associated with it.

In reducing symptoms, **drugs never create new functions.** They can only stimulate or depress the functions already inherent in the cells. Oral hypoglycemic agents stimulate the pancreas but not the kidney to release insulin.

In alleviating symptoms, drugs may also induce adverse effects, which may or may not be acceptable to patients. For instance, numerous agents with anticholinergic properties cause dry mouth, which is easily correctable and hence is acceptable to patients. Conversely, some antihypertensive medications cause impotence in male patients, which they may find unacceptable, and this side effect may thus lead to lack of compliance with the prescribed drug regimen.

It is clear that drugs resemble the proverbial double-edged sword, being able to help or hurt the patient further. By fully appreciating the nature of pharmacokinetics, pharmacodynamic principles, and drug-drug interactions, practitioners can drastically reduce unwanted side effects and at the same time enhance the therapeutic efficacy and usefulness of drugs in alleviating the mental and physical suffering of their patients.

I

Principles of Pharmacology

Notice

The indications and dosages of all drugs in this book have been recommended in the medical literature and conform to the practices of the general medical community. The medications described do not necessarily have specific approval by the Food and Drug Administration for use in the diseases and dosages for which they are recommended. The package insert for each drug should be consulted for use and dosage as approved by the FDA. Because standards for usage change, it is advisable to keep abreast of revised recommendations, particularly those concerning new drugs.

CHAPTER 1

The Pharmacokinetic Basis of Therapeutics

The primary objectives of therapy are to prevent or cure disease. The secondary objective, if these goals are not achievable, is to use drugs that mitigate the progressive, devastating, or disabling aspects of disease. The nature of the disease then determines the amount of drug or drugs to be given and the duration of therapy.

Pharmacokinetic principles deal with the **absorption, distribution, binding, biotransformation,** and **excretion** of drugs and their metabolites in the body. ■ **Fig. 1-1** ■

Administration of Drugs

Drugs are administered as a **solid** (in the form of capsules, tablets, or pills), a **volatile liquid,** a **solution,** an **aerosol,** a **gas,** or a **crystalline suspension.** The route of administration is chosen based on the desired onset and duration of action of the drug, the nature of the drug, any special circumstances, and the bioavailability of the drug.

Bioavailability

The physiochemical nature of certain drugs may rule out oral administration, and hence these drugs are considered to have subnormal oral bioavailability. For example, nitroglycerin is given sublingually in the treatment of angina pectoris because it is catabolized very rapidly in the liver if it is given orally.

Absorption of Drugs

The various lipoid barriers of the GI tract, the kidney tubules, and the CNS allow the absorption of essential nutrients, guard against the uncontrollable disposal of electrolytes and other substances, and prevent the entrance of potentially toxic materials.

To reach its site of action (the **receptor**), a drug may have to traverse a succession of membranes.

Multiple **physical and chemical factors** influence the rate and extent of absorption of drugs:

Physiochemical factors
Molecular weight
Degree of ionization under physiologic conditions
Product formulation characteristics
Disintegration and dissolution rates for solid dosages
Drug-release characteristics for timed-release preparations

Patient factors
Surface area available for absorption
Gastric and duodenal pHs
Gastric emptying time
Bile salt pool size
Bacterial colonization of the GI tract
Presence and extent of underlying diseases

Lipid-soluble substances traverse the membrane by dissolving in the lipoid phase, and lipid-insoluble substances penetrate only when they are small enough to pass through the pores. The absorption of large lipid-insoluble substances such as sugars and amino acids is accomplished by **specialized transport processes.**

Transport Mechanisms

Passive Diffusion - Passive diffusion takes place when a drug molecule moves from a region of relatively high to low concentration without requiring energy.

Carrier-Mediated Transport - A substance to be carried forms a complex with a component of the membrane on one side. The complex is then carried through the membrane, the drug or substance is released, and the carrier returns to the original surface or state, to repeat the process.

Facilitated Transport - Facilitated transport is essentially the same as carrier-mediated transport except that a transport facilitator in addition to a carrier molecule is essential. For example, vitamin B_{12} attaches to the **intrinsic factor,** and the vitamin B_{12}–intrinsic factor complex then attaches to the car-

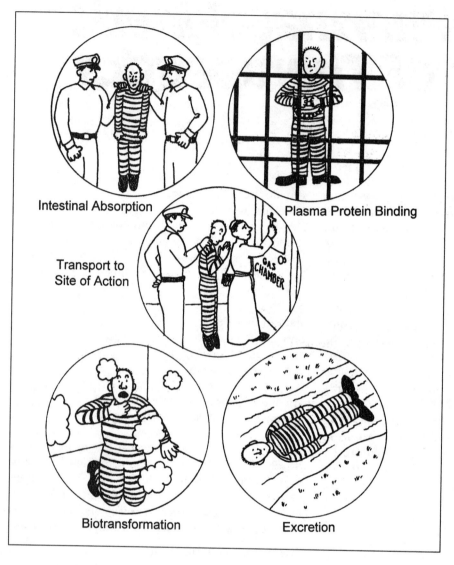

Intestinal Absorption

Plasma Protein Binding

Transport to
Site of Action

Biotransformation

Excretion

■ **Fig. 1-1** ■
Principles of
pharmacokinetics.

rier molecule and is transported. This transport process does not require energy and does not proceed against a concentration gradient.

Pinocytosis

In pinocytosis, the transport of water-insoluble substances such as **vitamins A, D, E,** and **K** is accomplished in the following manner. First the substances are engulfed by the membranes. Then they are dissolved in the membranes and released unchanged in the inside compartment.

Receptor-Mediated Endocytosis

Receptor-mediated endocytosis is the process of **ligand movement** from the extracellular space to the inside of the cell by the interaction of the ligand with a specific **cell-surface receptor.** Receptors bind the ligand at the surface, internalize it by means of coated

pits and vesicles, and ultimately release it into an acidic endosomal compartment.

Other Factors Controlling the Rate of Absorption of Drugs

In addition to the **lipid-water partition coefficient,** other factors that control the rate of absorption of drugs are the **degree of ionization,** the **surface area, blood flow** through the region, and the **gastric emptying time.**

Degree of Ionization - The **degree of dissociation** of drugs and the **pH of the internal medium** play important roles in the transfer of drugs across biologic membranes.

Surface Area - The influence of ionization on drug absorption is important only in circumstances in which biologic pHs vary dramatically, such as those in the stomach (varying from 1.4 to 7.0) and the urine (varying from 4.5 to 7.5). The changes in pH in other biologic fluids are considerably smaller. Because both ionized and nonionized drugs are absorbed from subcutaneous and intramuscular (IM) sites of injection, ionization does not appear to play as important a role in the passage of drugs across the capillary wall. Finally, although drugs such as acetylsalicylic acid are best absorbed from an acidic medium such as that in the stomach, most of the aspirin is nevertheless absorbed in the upper small intestine, which has a considerably greater absorptive surface. The **total absorptive area** of the small intestine and its microvilli has been estimated to exceed 200 m² for the intestine versus 1 m² for the stomach. Similarly, the **perfusion rate** of the intestine is considerably greater than that of the stomach. In fact, most drugs, whether nonionized or ionized and whether acidic, basic, or neutral, are absorbed mostly from the small intestine. Consistent with this is the observation that buffered acetylsalicylic acid preparations are dissolved faster and absorbed better mostly in the intestine. Similarly, patients with **achlorhydria** or those who have undergone gastrectomy have little difficulty with the absorption of orally ingested drugs.

Blood Flow - The absorption of drugs in solution from IM and subcutaneous sites of injection is limited by the **perfusion** rate.

Gastric Emptying Time - Because drugs are mostly absorbed from the upper part of the small intestine, the rate of gastric emptying plays a crucial role in drug absorption. If rapid absorption is desired, drugs should be taken on an empty stomach.

Hepatic First-Pass Effect

By far the most important reason for an inadequate plasma concentration following the oral or parenteral administration of a drug is the **first-pass effect,** which consists of the loss of a drug as it passes through the liver for the first time.

Distribution of Drugs

Whether given orally or parenterally, drugs are distributed nonuniformly throughout the body. Factors that regulate this distribution are the **lipophilic characteristics** of the drugs, the **blood supply** to the tissues, and the **chemical** composition of various organs and tissues. The distribution of drugs not only influences their **onset of action** but also at times determines their **duration of action.**

Binding of Various Drugs to Plasma Proteins

In an ideal therapeutic regimen, a sufficient amount of the drug should reach the locus of action (receptor site) in order to bring about the desired effect but not so much as to produce toxicity. Furthermore, the drug should not disappear too rapidly from the locus of action, or the therapeutic effects will be transient and hence of limited value. The binding of drugs to plasma proteins and various subcellular components tends to accomplish these objectives. ■ **Fig. 1-2** ■ A number of plasma proteins, especially albumin, have shown a high affinity for binding drugs, so that at a given total plasma concentration, only a portion of the total amount of drug is free in the plasma water. The remainder is bound to plasma proteins and in this form does not exert any pharmacologic effects.

Tissue Localization of Drugs

After a drug has been absorbed, the initial phase of its distribution into the tissues is based on **cardiac output** and **regional blood flow.** Highly perfused organs such as the brain, heart, liver, and kidney receive most of the drug. Diffusion into the interstitial compartment occurs rapidly. **Lipid-soluble** and **lipid-insoluble drugs** have different patterns of distribution; for example, thiopental, a highly lipid-soluble substance, distributes rapidly into the brain.

Apparent Volume of Distribution of Drugs

Volume of distribution (V_D) is defined as the amount of drug in the body in relation to the concentration of drug in the plasma:

$$V_D = \frac{\text{Amount of drug in body}}{\text{Concentration of drug in plasma}}$$

Blood-Brain Barrier

The brain capillaries are tightly joined and covered by a footlike sheath that arises from astrocytes. Thus, a drug leaving the capillaries in the brain has to traverse not only the nonporous capillary cell wall, but also the membranes of the astrocyte, in order to reach the neurons. Such a structure, frequently referred to as the **blood-brain barrier,** tends to limit the entry of many drugs into the brain.

Placental Barrier

The membrane separating fetal blood from maternal blood in the intervillous space, the **placental barrier,** resembles other membranes, in that lipid-soluble substances diffuse readily but water-soluble substances

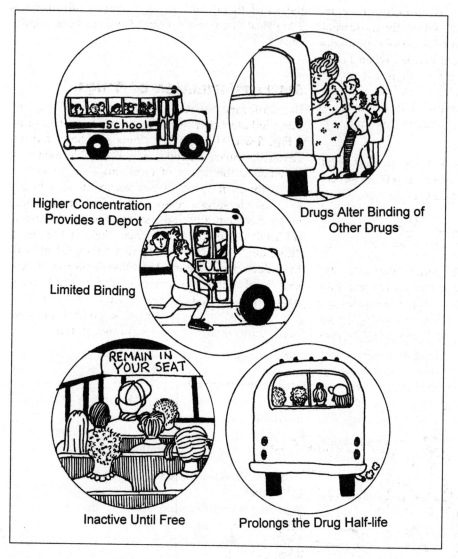

Higher Concentration
Provides a Depot

Drugs Alter Binding of
Other Drugs

Limited Binding

REMAIN IN
YOUR SEAT

Inactive Until Free

Prolongs the Drug Half-life

■ **Fig. 1-2** ■
Binding of drugs to plasma
proteins.

either do not diffuse or diffuse poorly. **Anesthetics** and **analgesics** readily cross both the blood-brain and placental barriers. Thus, for instance, morphine-induced respiratory depression and miosis may occur in both the mother and her newborn infant. The children of narcotic-addicted mothers will be born with an addiction to narcotics.

Site of Action of Drugs

It is generally accepted that most drugs exert their potent and specific effects by forming a bond, generally reversible, with a cellular component called a **receptor site.** Drugs that interact with a receptor and elicit a response are called **agonists.** Drugs that interact with receptors and prevent the action of agonists are termed **antagonists.** The relative effects of drugs are often judged in terms of their **potency,** a measure of the dosage required to bring about a re-

sponse, and their **efficacy,** a measure of their inherent ability to exert an effect.

Dose-Response Relationship

The relationship between the amount of drug administered (e.g., morphine), or the concentration of the administered drug in the plasma, and the magnitude of the desired response obtained (e.g., analgesia) is referred to as a **dose-response relationship.**

The interaction between a drug and a receptor site is similar to a reversible interaction between a substrate and an enzyme. This antagonism between agonists and antagonists is called **competitive** or **surmountable antagonism** if the inhibition is overcome by increasing the concentration of the agonist. For example, propranolol (a beta-adrenergic receptor antagonist) is a competitive antagonist for isoproterenol (a beta-adrenergic receptor agonist), and atropine is a competitive antagonist for acetylcholine at the muscarinic cholinergic receptor site. A **partial agonist** produces a lower response than a full agonist does. When a maximum response is obtained by an agonist at a concentration that does not occupy all the available receptor, a **spare receptor** or high-efficacy receptor-agonist occupancy mechanism may be involved.

Therapeutic Index

The therapeutic index deals with the ratio of lethal doses to 50 percent of the population (LD_{50}) over the median minimum effective dose (ED_{50}):

$$\text{Therapeutic index} = \frac{LD_{50}}{ED_{50}}$$

The higher the therapeutic index, the safer the drug; the lower the therapeutic index, the greater the possibility of toxicity. The therapeutic index for barbiturates as a class is 10, whereas the therapeutic index for cardiac glycosides as a class is 3. Because

the usual therapeutic dose of cardiac glycoside is 1 mg, death may result if only 3 mg has been administered.

Biotransformation of Drugs

Biotransformation may be defined as the enzyme-catalyzed alteration of drugs by the living organism. ■ **Fig. 1-3** ■ Although few drugs are eliminated unchanged, urinary excretion is a negligible means of terminating the action of most drugs or poisons in the body. In fact, the urinary excretion of a highly lipid-soluble substance such as pentobarbital would be so slow that it would take the body a century to rid itself of the effect of a single dose of the agent. Therefore, mammalian and other terrestrial animals have developed systems that allow the conversion of most lipid-soluble substances to water-soluble ones, so that they may be easily excreted by the kidney. In general, biotransformation may be divided into two, hepatic and nonhepatic forms of metabolism.

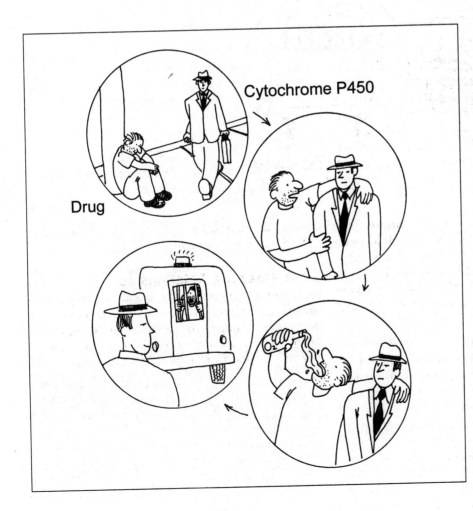

■ **Fig. 1-3** ■
Mechanism of action of cytochrome P-450.

Hepatic Drug Metabolism

By far the major portion of biotransformation is carried out in the liver by **cytochrome P-450** (P-450), which is a collective term for a group of related enzymes or isoenzymes that are responsible for the oxidation of numerous drugs; **endogenous substances** such as fatty acids, prostaglandins, steroids, and ketones; and **carcinogens** such as polycyclic aromatic hydrocarbons, nitrosamines, hydrazines, and arylamines. See ■ **Fig. 1-3** ■

During **Phase I**, most drugs are inactivated pharmacologically; some remain unaltered, and some become more active and toxic. For example, phenytoin in the liver is first hydroxylated to hydroxyphenytoin (Phase I) and is then conjugated with glucuronic acid (**Phase II**) and excreted by the kidney as phenytoin glucuronide conjugate. During Phase I, besides introducing a polar group such as an –OH group, a potential polar group may also be unmasked from the drug to be metabolized. For example, compound R–OCH$_3$ is converted to compound R–OH by demethylation. Codeine becomes demethylated to morphine. The free or unmasked polar group is then conjugated with glucuronate, sulfate, glycine, or acetate. With the exception of morphine 6-glucuronide, almost all conjugates lack pharmacologic activity.

Scheme of the Mixed-Function Oxidation Reaction Pathway

- The hepatic endoplasmic reticulum possesses oxidative enzymes called **mixed-function oxidases** or **monooxygenase** with a specific requirement for both molecular oxygen and a reduced concentration of nicotinamide adenine dinucleotide phosphate (NADPH). Essential in the mixed-function oxidase system is P-450. The primary electron donor is NADPH, whereas the electron transfer involves P-450, a flavoprotein. The presence of a **heat-stable fraction** is necessary for the operation of the system. See ■ **Fig. 1-3** ■

A drug substrate to be metabolized binds to oxidized P-450, which is reduced by P-450 reductase. The drug-reduced P-450 complex then combines with molecular oxygen. A second electron and two hydrogen ions are acquired from the donor system, and the subsequent products are oxidized drug and water, with regeneration of the oxidized P-450. This process ■ **Fig. 1-3** ■ is summarized as follows:

1. NADPH + oxidized cytochrome P-450 + H$^+$ → reduced P-450 + NADP$^+$
2. Reduced cytochrome P-450 + O$_2$ → "active oxygen complex"
3. "Active oxygen complex" + drug substrate → oxidized drug + oxidized cytochrome P-450 + H$_2$O

NADPH + O$_2$ + drug substrate + H$^+$ → NADP$^+$ + oxidized drug + H$_2$O

Nonhepatic Metabolism

Among the nonhepatic drug-metabolizing systems, only those in the intestinal epithelium, lung, and plasma have been studied.

Factors Modifying the Metabolism of Drugs

Many environmental factors and pathophysiologic conditions inhibit or stimulate the activity of drug-metabolizing enzymes, and hence may alter the outcome of a therapeutic regimen. Pharmacogenetics, the immaturity of drug-metabolizing enzyme systems, and drug-drug interactions are a few of the factors that can alter drug metabolism.

Pharmacogenetics

- Pharmacogenetics represents the study of the hereditary variation in the handling of drugs. Pharmacogenetic abnormalities may be entirely innocuous, until the affected individual is challenged with particular drugs.

Liver Disease

- The liver is the principal metabolic organ, and hepatic disease or dysfunction may impair drug elimination. Any alteration in the serum albumin or bilirubin levels and in the prothrombin time indicates impaired liver function. Similarly, skin bruising and bleeding tendency indicate decreased production of clotting factors by the liver.

The Influence of Age

- Drug metabolism is qualitatively and quantitatively very deficient in **newborns.** For example, **chloramphenicol,** when used injudiciously, may cause **gray syndrome.** The **elderly** are also prone to toxicity from numerous drugs, including cardiac glycosides. A dose of digitoxin that may be totally therapeutic and innocuous to someone aged 60 may produce severe toxicity and even death at the age of 70. The abilities of the liver to metabolize drugs and the kidney to excrete drug metabolites decline with aging.

Enzyme Induction and Inhibition

- The activities of **microsomal drug-metabolizing enzymes** in humans can be enhanced by altering the levels of endogenous hormones such as androgens, estrogens, progestational steroids, glucocorticoids, anabolic steroids, norepinephrine, insulin, and thyroxine. This effect can also be elicited by the administration of exogenous substances such as drugs, food preservatives, insecticides, herbicides, and polycyclic aromatic hydrocarbons. This increase in the activities of drug-metabolizing enzymes appears to stem from an elevated rate of synthesis of the enzyme protein; hence, it is truly an enzyme-induction phenomenon.

Clinical Implications of Enzyme Induction and Inhibition - Patients are often given several drugs at the same time. The possibility that one drug may accelerate or inhibit the metabolism of another drug should always be kept in mind. When this phenomenon occurs, the removal of an enzyme inducer could be hazardous.

Excretion of Drugs

An orally administered drug will gradually begin to be absorbed. As the amount of drug in the body increases by 50%, the amount of the drug at the absorption site should decrease by the same amount. The absorbed drug will gradually be metabolized or excreted mostly by the kidneys. See ■ **Fig. 1-1** ■

Rate of Excretion of Drugs by the Kidneys

The amount of a drug (or its metabolites) that appears in the urine depends on the amount of drug undergoing **glomerular filtration, tubular secretion,** and **tubular resorption.** Metabolism plays a major role in drug excretion, since the metabolites are more water-soluble substances, which are excreted. Drugs are excreted when they are in their free form, but plasma protein-bound drugs and tissue-stored drugs are not excreted.

The excretion of drugs from the kidneys, like the absorption of drugs from the GI tract, depends on lipid solubility, the degree of ionization of drugs, and the pH of the urine. Nonionized lipid-soluble drugs are resorbed and not eliminated. Generally drugs that are bases are excreted when the urine is acidic, whereas acidic compounds are excreted in greater quantities if the urine is alkaline. For example, in **phenobarbital** (weak acid pK_a of 7.3) poisoning, alkalinization of the urine with sodium bicarbonate is helpful in eliminating the phenobarbital. In **amphetamine** toxicity, acidification of the urine with ammonium chloride is required.

Drugs that undergo both glomerular filtration and active tubular secretion have a very short half-life. **Penicillin** is one such compound, but its half-life is prolonged by the coadministration of **probenecid,** a uricosuric drug that inhibits the tubular secretion of penicillin. Most drugs, however, have half-lives that are relatively longer than penicillin's because they undergo glomerular filtration, partial tubular resorption, and no active tubular secretion.

Significance of Blood Flow on Drug Clearance

In general, the rate of extraction of drug from blood and the rate of clearance by the kidney depend on blood flow and the ability of the kidney to extract the drug (the **extraction ratio**). If all of the drug is removed from the blood as it traverses through the kidneys, the extraction ratio is 1. The higher the blood flow is, the higher is the rate of excretion of that drug; and the clearance is said to be **perfusion-rate limited.** For example, the extraction ratio of digoxin, one of the cardiac glycosides, is low, and toxicity is likely to occur in renal failure. Similarly, the hepatic extraction ratio of digitoxin is low, and toxicity is likely to occur in hepatic failure. Consequently, cardiologists have long recognized that **digitoxin** and **digoxin** should be avoided in patients suffering from liver and renal failure, respectively.

Half-Life of a Drug

The half-life of a drug, or its elimination half-life, is the time required for its concentration in the blood to be reduced by one-half. For penicillin G, the half-life is 20 minutes, indicating that only 50% of it remains in the blood 20 minutes after its IV administration. Both the IV and orally administered identical drugs have the same half-lives once they reach the general circulation. When given at regular intervals, a drug or its metabolite reaches a certain plateau concentration after approximately four to five half-lives. This plateau changes only if the dose or frequency of administration, or both, are altered.

CHAPTER 2

Pharmacodynamics

Pharmacodynamics is the study of the actions and effects of drugs on organ, tissue, cellular, and subcellular levels. It provides information about how drugs bring about their beneficial effects and how they cause their side effects.

Site of Action

The receptor sites where a drug acts to initiate a group of functions is that drug's site of action. The central sites of action of morphine, for example, are the cerebral cortex, hypothalamus, and medullary center.

Mode of Action

The character of an effect produced by a drug is called the **mode of action** of that drug. Morphine, by depressing the function of the cerebral cortex, hypothalamus, and medullary center, is responsible for decreasing pain perception (analgesia), inducing narcosis (heavy sedation), depressing the cough center (antitussive effect), initially stimulating and then depressing the vomiting center, and depressing respiration.

Mechanism of Action

The identification of molecular and biochemical events leading to an effect is called the **mechanism of action** of that drug. For instance, morphine causes respiratory depression by depressing the responsiveness of the respiratory center to carbon dioxide.

Cellular Sites of Action of Drugs

Because drugs are very reactive, they may elicit their effects or side effects, or both, by interacting with coenzymes, enzymes, or nucleic acids, as well as other macromolecules and physiologic processes, such as transport mechanisms. Some examples will point out the complex interactions between drugs and physiologic parameters.

Drug-Coenzyme Interactions

The primary drugs that combine the greatest level of efficacy with an acceptable degree of toxicity in the treatment of **tuberculosis** are isoniazid, ethambutol, pyrazinamide, and rifampin. **Isoniazid** is prescribed orally in doses of 4–5 mg/kg of body weight. If pyridoxine is not given with the isoniazid, peripheral neuritis is the most common side effect. In toxic doses, optic neuritis, muscular twitching, dizziness, ataxia, paresthesias, and convulsions may occur, especially in malnourished patients. These neuropathies are thought to result from a chemical interaction between isoniazid and **pyridoxal phosphate** and the reduced level of this important coenzyme in the body. The coadministration of pyridoxine averts these side effects.

Drug-Enzyme Interaction

Numerous drugs exert their effects and side effects by interacting with enzymes. **Allopurinol** is used to lower uric acid levels in the treatment of primary gout, as a prophylaxis in myeloproliferative neoplastic disease, for investigational purposes in Lesch-Nyhan syndrome, and as an adjunct with thiazide diuretics or ethambutol. The mechanism of action of allopurinol is the inhibition of xanthine oxidase, which converts hypoxanthine into xanthine and in turn becomes oxidized into uric acid:

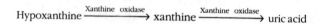

$$\text{Hypoxanthine} \xrightarrow{\text{Xanthine oxidase}} \text{xanthine} \xrightarrow{\text{Xanthine oxidase}} \text{uric acid}$$

When xanthine oxidase is inhibited by allopurinol, the plasma level of uric acid and the size of the urate pool in the body decrease.

Drug–Nucleic Acid Interactions

Chemotherapeutic agents useful in the treatment of neoplastic diseases exert their therapeutic effects by modifying the synthesis or functions of nucleic acids.

For example, **6-mercaptopurine** inhibits purine-ring biosynthesis, **cytarabine** inhibits DNA polymerase, **alkylating agents** crosslink DNA, and **hydroxyurea** inhibits the conversion of ribonucleotides into deoxyribonucleotides.

Interactions of Drugs with Neuronal Elements

Neuropharmacology is the study of drugs that affect the nervous system and its neuronal components. The functions of the nervous system are intimately linked with the synthesis, storage, release, and uptake of many transmitters and their modulators. The beneficial effects or side effects of an extensive number of drugs are brought about through their interaction with these neurotransmitter-neuromodulator systems.

Interaction of Drugs with the Endocrine System

Hypotension and decreased renal perfusion pressure promote the release of renin from the juxtaglomerular apparatus of the kidney. **Renin** converts angiotensin I to **angiotensin II,** a potent endogenously occurring vasoconstrictor. Catecholamine can also release renin, and this effect is blocked by **propranolol,** a beta-adrenergic receptor blocking agent. Drugs that alter the renin level can alter blood pressure. **Alpha-methyldopa** suppresses renin release, whereas oral contraceptives have the opposite effect. In addition, other antihypertensive medications such as **captopril** inhibit angiotensin-converting enzyme, hence preventing the formation of angiotensin II.

Drugs do not create functions but merely stimulate or inhibit functions already inherent in the cells. These pharmacodynamic-related interactions take place at various levels of cellular activities, including ion transport, enzymes, coenzymes, nucleic acids, and numerous other biochemical events yet to be delineated.

CHAPTER 3

Adverse Reactions and Drug-Drug Interactions

On medical services, it is common for patients with **multiple medical problems** to take as many as 10 to 15 drugs concomitantly. It is also becoming increasingly obvious to physicians and other members of the healthcare delivery team that many **drug combinations,** when used inappropriately and injudiciously, have the inherent potential to interact adversely, leading to side effects and even death. ■ **Fig. 3-1** ■

Iatrogenic Reactions

Iatrogenic reactions are adverse reactions produced unintentionally by physicians in their patients. For example, one of the side effects of many antihistaminic preparations (H_1 antagonists) such as ethanolamine derivatives (prototype: diphenhydramine) is heavy sedation.

Allergic Reactions

Drug allergy refers to those drug reactions in a patient who was previously exposed to, sensitized with, and developed antibodies to a drug. ■ **Fig. 3-1** ■

Idiosyncratic Reactions

Idiosyncrasy refers to an abnormal, unexpected, or peculiar reaction seen in only certain patients. For example, **succinylcholine** may cause prolonged apnea in patients with **pseudocholinesterase deficiency.** See ■ **Fig. 3-1** ■

Tolerance and Tachyphylaxis

Tolerance refers to decreased responses following the long-term administration of drugs. For example, after repeated **morphine** use, tolerance to all of its effects occurs, except for miosis and constipation, which continue.

Tachyphylaxis refers to a quickly developing tolerance brought about by the rapid and repeated administration of drugs. For example, indirect-acting sympathomimetic agents such as **tyramine,** which exert their effects through the release of norepinephrine, can cause tachyphylaxis. If norepinephrine is not present, tyramine fails to exert its effect until the supply of norepinephrine in nerve terminals has been replenished.

Supersensitivity

Supersensitivity refers to increased responsiveness to a drug that results either from denervation or following administration of a drug (a receptor antagonist) for a prolonged period of time.

Pharmacokinetic Interactions

Drugs may affect the absorption, distribution, metabolism, or excretion of other drugs. This includes those interactions in which the GI absorption of a drug, plasma protein binding, drug metabolism, and urinary excretion are either enhanced or inhibited. ■ **Fig. 3-2** ■

Interaction at the Site of Absorption

The rate or extent of drug absorption from the GI tract can be influenced in a number of ways. Following are examples of these various influences.

Alteration of Gastric pH

Deferoxamine, which binds iron, is the preferred chelator in treating **iron poisoning**. The metabolic acidosis caused by iron poisoning may be appropriately treated with sodium bicarbonate. However, because deferoxamine chelates iron more effectively in an acidic medium, it should not be administered orally along with sodium bicarbonate.

Formation of Complex

The absorption of **tetracyclines** is hindered by milk and milk products; by numerous **antacids** such as aluminum hydroxide, sodium bicarbonate, and

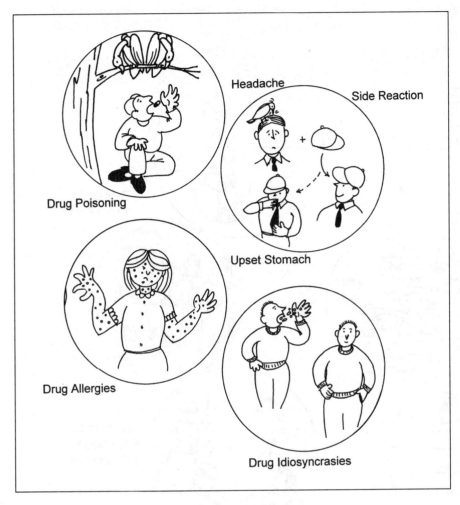

Headache

Side Reaction

Drug Poisoning

Upset Stomach

Drug Allergies

Drug Idiosyncrasies

■ **Fig. 3-1** ■
Interactions among drugs.

calcium carbonate; and by iron preparations such as ferrous sulfate.

Alteration in Gastric Emptying Time

Agents that reduce GI motility and prolong gastric emptying time reduce the rate of absorption of drugs whose absorption takes place primarily in the duodenum.

Interactions at the Plasma Protein-Binding Sites

Drugs may **compete** for binding sites on the plasma or tissue protein, or they may **displace** previously bound drugs. For example, **phenylbutazone** may compete with **phenytoin** for binding to albumin. See ■ **Fig. 3-2** ■

Interactions at the Stage of Drug Biotransformation

Drug biotransformation usually converts the nonpolar active drugs into more water-soluble but pharmacologically inactive products. Drugs may stimulate or inhibit the metabolism of other drugs. See ■ **Fig. 3-2** ■

Interactions at the Site of Excretion

Numerous drugs either enhance or inhibit the excretion of other drugs. For example, **sodium bicarbonate** enhances the excretion of **phenobarbital.** Probenecid interferes with the active secretion of penicillin and hence prolongs its half-life. Probenecid's uricosuric effects are counteracted by acetylsalicylic acid, which also possesses a uricosuric effect. When given concomitantly, both are excreted. See ■ **Fig. 3-2** ■

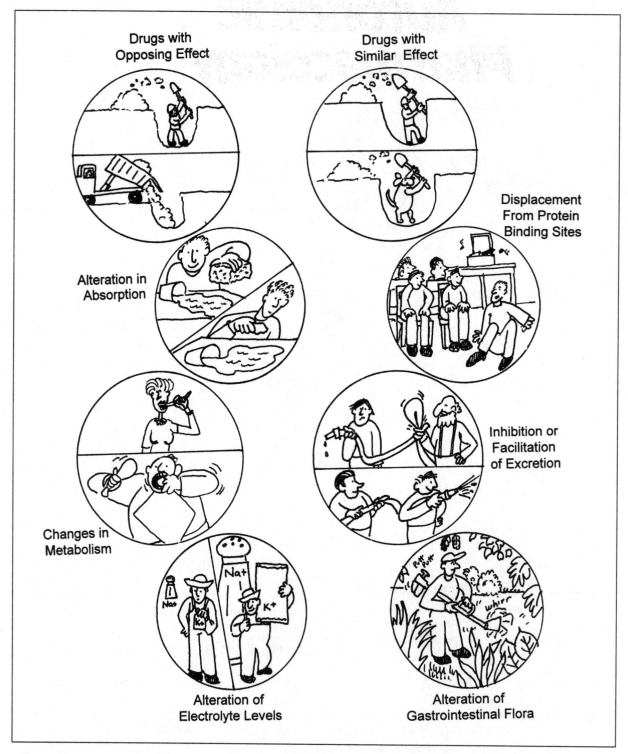

■ **Fig. 3-2** ■
Drug toxicity.

II

Autonomic Pharmacology

CHAPTER 4

The Autonomic Nervous System

The nervous and endocrine systems control an extensive number of functions in the body. The nervous system is divided into the **central nervous system** (CNS) and the **peripheral nervous system.** The peripheral nervous system is further divided into the **somatic nervous system** (a voluntary system innervating skeletal muscles) and the **autonomic nervous system** (an involuntary system innervating smooth muscle, cardiac muscle, and glands). ■ **Fig. 4-1** ■

Autonomic Drugs

Autonomic drugs have extensive clinical applications. They are used in the treatment of wide-angle glaucoma, in the diagnosis of myasthenia gravis, as a GI and urinary tract stimulant in postoperative abdominal distention and urinary retention, as antidotes to poisoning from curare and the tricyclic antidepressants, as preanesthetic medications, as mydriatics, as cycloplegics, in peptic acid oversecretion to diminish the vagally mediated secretion of gastric juices, in slowing of gastric emptying, in vestibular disorders, in parkinsonism, in combination with local anesthetics, in hypotension and shock, in heart block to improve atrioventricular conduction and stimulate ventricular automaticity, in bronchial asthma, as a nasal decongestant, in narcolepsy, in attention deficit hyperactivity disorders, in the diagnosis and treatment of pheochromocytoma, in cardiac arrhythmias, in angina pectoris, in hypertension, in thyrotoxicosis, and in tremor. In addition, numerous drugs such as neuroleptics and antidepressants produce side effects by modifying the functions of the autonomic nervous system.

Division and Functions of the Autonomic Nervous System

The autonomic nervous system is divided into two major portions: the **sympathetic (thoracolumbar)** division and the **parasympathetic (craniosacral)** division. See ■ **Fig. 4-1** ■ Both divisions originate in nuclei within the CNS and give rise to preganglionic efferent fibers that exit from the brainstem or spinal cord and terminate in motor ganglia. A large number of peripheral autonomic nervous system fibers synthesize and release acetylcholine. These include all preganglionic efferent autonomic fibers and the somatic motor fibers to skeletal muscles. Most postganglionic sympathetic fibers release norepinephrine. See ■ **Fig. 4-1** ■

Cholinergic Transmission

Neurochemical Basis of Cholinergic Transmission

Acetylcholine, an ester of choline and acetic acid, is synthesized in cholinergic neurons according to the following scheme:

$$\text{Acetyl coenzyme A + choline} \xrightarrow{\text{Choline acetyltransferase}} \text{acetylcholine}$$

The acetylcholine, in turn, is hydrolyzed by both **acetylcholinesterase** and plasma butyrylcholinesterase. **Choline** is actively transported into nerve terminals (synaptosomes) by a high-affinity uptake mechanism. Furthermore, the availability of choline regulates the synthesis of acetylcholine. ■ **Fig. 4-2** ■

Hemicholinium blocks the transport of choline into synaptosomes, whereas **botulinum toxin** blocks the calcium-mediated release of acetylcholine. ■ **Fig. 4-3** ■ The released acetylcholine is hydrolyzed rapidly by acetylcholinesterase to choline and acetate.

Classification of Cholinergic Receptors

Acetylcholine receptors are classified as either **muscarinic** or **nicotinic.** The alkaloid **muscarine** mimics the effects produced by stimulation of the parasympathetic system. These effects are postganglionic and are exerted on exocrine glands, cardiac muscle, and smooth muscle. The alkaloid **nicotine**

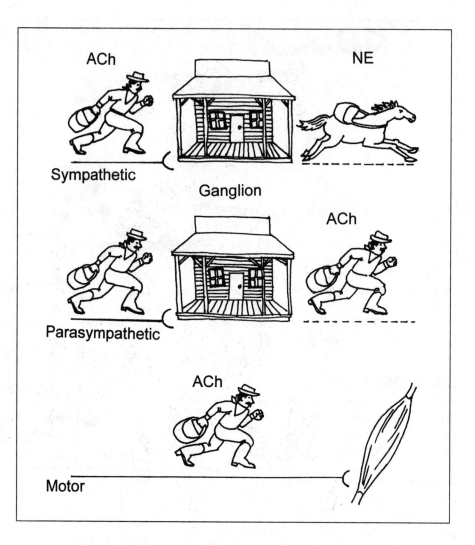

■ Fig. 4-1 ■

Neurotransmitters of the autonomic nervous system.

mimics the actions of acetylcholine, which include stimulation of all autonomic ganglia, stimulation of the adrenal medulla, and contraction of skeletal muscle.

Dimethylphenylpiperazinium stimulates the autonomic ganglia, **tetraethylammonium** and **hexamethonium** block the autonomic ganglia, **phenyltrimethylammonium** stimulates skeletal motor muscle end plates, **decamethonium** produces neuromuscular blockade, and **d-tubocurarine** blocks both the autonomic ganglia and the motor fiber end plates. **■ Fig. 4-4 ■**

Cholinergic (Cholionimetic) Receptor Agonists

Methacholine, carbachol, and bethanechol are all agents that mimic the effects of stimulation of cholinergic nerves.

The two currently used derivatives of acetylcholine are **bethanechol** (urecholine chloride) and **carba-**

chol (Miostat). Unlike acetylcholine, both agents are resistant to hydrolysis by cholinesterase. Both agents are muscarinic agonists. The **nicotinic action** of carbachol is greater than that of acetylcholine, whereas bethanechol is devoid of nicotinic action. The **cardiovascular actions** of acetylcholine are vasodilation and negative chronotropic and inotropic effects. The cardiovascular effects of **methacholine** are more pronounced than those of acetylcholine, which in turn are greater than those of carbachol or bethanechol. The **GI effects** (increase in tone, amplitude of contractions, and peristalsis) of bethanechol and carbachol are equal but greater than those of acetylcholine. The effects of carbachol and bethanechol on the **urinary tract,** consisting of ureteral peristalsis, contraction of the detrusor muscle of the urinary bladder, and an increase in voluntary voiding pressure, are equivalent and exceed those produced by acetylcholine.

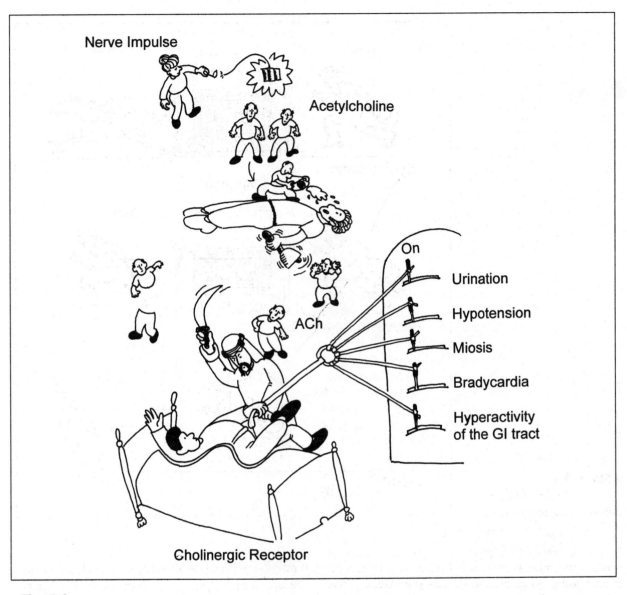

■ Fig. 4-2 ■
Synthesis, release, and actions of acetylcholine.

The **miotic effects** of carbachol and bethanechol are greater than those of acetylcholine.

Atropine is able to antagonize all cholinergic (muscarinic) effects produced by acetylcholine, methacholine, carbachol, and bethanechol. However, this antagonism is least evident with carbachol.

Bethanechol is of value in the management of postoperative abdominal distention, gastric atony or stasis, and urinary retention. Carbachol (0.25–3.0%) may be used for the long-term therapy of noncongestive wide-angle glaucoma.

Pilocarpine is a naturally occurring cholinomimetic agent possessing both muscarinic and nicotinic properties (stimulates autonomic ganglia). This agent causes miosis, reduces intraocular pressure, and is used in the treatment of wide-angle glaucoma. In addition, it may be applied topically in the eye in the form of a drug reservoir (Ocusert).

Anticholinesterase Agents

Anticholinesterases are drugs that inhibit or inactivate acetylcholinesterase, causing the accumulation of acetylcholine at the cholinergic receptors. **■ Fig. 4-5 ■**

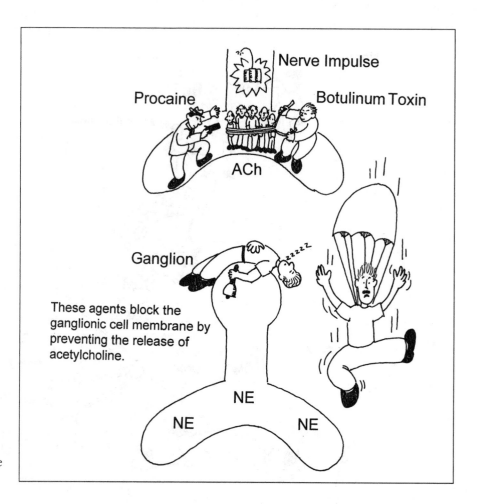

Nerve Impulse

Procaine

Botulinum Toxin

ACh

Ganglion

These agents block the
ganglionic cell membrane by
preventing the release of
acetylcholine.

NE

NE   NE

■ Fig. 4-3 ■
Botulinus toxin prevents the
release of acetylcholine.

Classification of Cholinesterase Inhibitors

The **reversible inhibitors,** which have a short to
moderate duration of action, fall into two categories.
Type one, exemplified by **edrophonium,** forms
an ionic bond at the anionic site and a weak hydrogen bond at the esteratic site of acetylcholinesterase.
Type two, exemplified by **neostigmine,** forms an
ionic bond at the anionic site and a hydrolyzable covalent bond at the esteratic site. **■ Fig. 4-5 ■**

The **irreversible inhibitors,** exemplified by organophosphorous compounds (diisopropylfluorophosphate
[DFP], parathion, malathion, diazinon), have long du-
rations of action and form a covalent bond with
acetylcholinesterase, which is hydrolyzed very slowly
and negligibly, but the inhibition may be overcome
by cholinesterase activators such as pralidoxime (PAM).
■ Fig. 4-6 ■

Cholinesterase inhibitors may also be classified according to agents that possess **tertiary nitrogens** (e.g.,
physostigmine and most organophosphorous com-

pounds) and those that contain **quaternary nitrogens**
(e.g., neostigmine, pyridostigmine, and some organophosphorous compounds such as echothiophate).
■ Table 4-1 ■ summarizes the comparative properties of these agents.

Physostigmine (eserine sulfate) causes miosis and
spasm of accommodation; it also lowers intraocular
pressure and hence can be used in the treatment of
wide-angle glaucoma. Being lipid soluble, it penetrates into the brain rapidly, raises the acetylcholine
concentration, and in toxic amounts may cause
cholinergic CNS toxicity, which is characterized by
restlessness, insomnia, tremors, confusion, ataxia,
convulsions, respiratory depression, and circulatory
collapse. These effects are reversed by atropine.

Neostigmine, which is unable to penetrate the blood-
brain barrier, does not cause CNS toxicity. However, it
may produce a dose-dependent and full range of
muscarinic effects, characterized by miosis, blurring
of vision, lacrimation, salivation, sweating, increased
bronchial secretion, bronchoconstriction, bradycar-

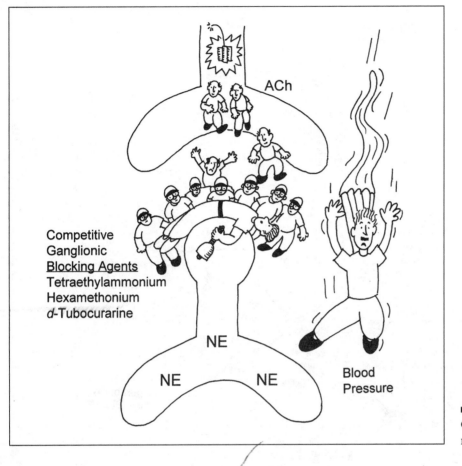

ACh

Competitive
Ganglionic
Blocking Agents
Tetraethylammonium
Hexamethonium
d-Tubocurarine

NE

NE   NE

Blood
Pressure

■ **Fig. 4-4** ■
Ganglionic blocking agents
may cause hypotension.

dia, hypotension, and urinary incontinence. Atropine is able to oppose these muscarinic effects. In addition, neostigmine, which has both a direct action and an indirect action that is mediated by acetylcholine on end-plate nicotinic receptors, may produce muscular fasciculation, muscular cramps, weakness, and even paralysis. These effects are not countered by atropine. Furthermore, neostigmine enhances gastric contraction and secretion. Neostigmine itself is metabolized by plasma acetylcholinesterase.

The therapeutic uses of neostigmine include the treatment of atony of the urinary bladder and postoperative abdominal distention. In addition, it antagonizes the action of *d*-tubocurarine and curariform drugs. Edrophonium, neostigmine, or pyridostigmine may be used to diagnose myasthenia gravis. Because edrophonium has the shortest duration of action, it is most often used for this purpose.

Antidote to Irreversible Cholinesterase Inhibitors

The irreversible cholinesterase inhibitors, such as **diiopropylfluorophosphate** (DFP, isofluorophate),

are used only for local application in the treatment of wide-angle glaucoma. Their pharmacologic effects, similar to those produced by physostigmine, are intense and of long duration. As **organophosphorous insecticides,** they are of paramount importance in cases of accidental poisoning and suicidal and homicidal attempts. They produce a **cholinergic crisis** that must be treated by (1) decontaminating the patient, (2) supporting respiration, (3) blocking the muscarinic effects by atropine, and (4) reactivating the inhibited cholinesterase by treatment with pralidoxime. See PAM in ■ **Fig. 4-6** ■

Cholinergic Receptor Blocking Agents

Atropine and **scopolamine,** as well as other synthetic anticholinergic drugs, inhibit the actions of acetylcholine and cholinomimetic drugs at muscarinic receptors in smooth muscles, heart, and exocrine glands. ■ **Fig. 4-7** ■ In addition to these peripheral effects, anticholinergic drugs, by blocking the acetylcholine receptor sites in the CNS, have pronounced

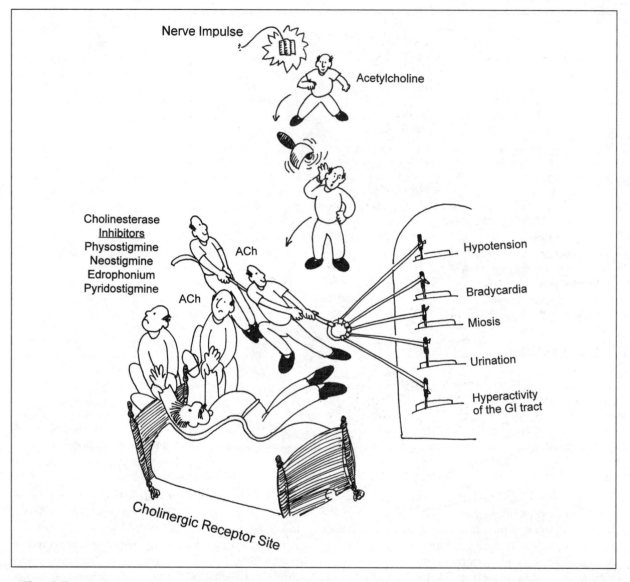

Nerve Impulse

Acetylcholine

Cholinesterase
Inhibitors
Physostigmine
Neostigmine
Edrophonium
Pyridostigmine

ACh

ACh

Hypotension

Bradycardia

Miosis

Urination

Hyperactivity
of the GI tract

Cholinergic Receptor Site

■ **Fig. 4-5** ■
Actions of cholinesterase inhibitors.

CNS effects, such as restlessness, irritability, excitement, and hallucinations. Scopolamine, on the other hand, depresses the CNS and in therapeutic doses produces fatigue, hypnosis, and amnesia. Therefore, it is used extensively in numerous medications, often in combination with antihistamines.

Dose-Dependent Effects of Atropine

The pharmacologic effects of atropine in general are dose dependent. For example, in small doses, atropine depresses sweating, elevates body temperature, decreases salivary and bronchial secretions, and relaxes

bronchial smooth muscles. In somewhat larger doses (1–3 mg), it produces mydriasis (blockade of the iris sphincter muscle), cycloplegia (blockade of the ciliary muscle), and cardiovascular effects characterized by transient bradycardia (central vagal stimulation) and tachycardia (vagal blockade at the sinoatrial node). Lacking any significant effects on circulation, atropine is often used as a preanesthetic medication to depress bronchial secretion and prevent pronounced bradycardia during abdominal surgical procedures. In still larger doses, it depresses the tone and motility of the GI tract, the tone of the urinary bladder, and

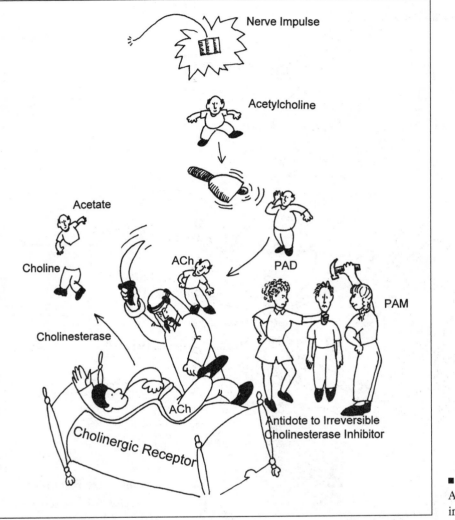

Fig. 4-6
Antidotes to cholinesterase inhibitors.

Table 4-1 Comparative Properties of Physostigmine and Neostigmine

	Physostigmine	Neostigmine
Oral absorption	Good	Poor
Passing across the blood-brain barrier	Well	No
Stimulating nicotinic receptors (skeletal muscle)	Yes	Yes
Used to combat the CNS toxicity of numerous anticholinergic drugs	Yes	No

gastric secretion. Therefore, the effective doses for use in acid-pepsin diseases are preceded by numerous side effects.

Atropine is absorbed orally and crosses the placental barrier, whereupon it causes fetal tachycardia. Atropine has been used to examine the functional integrity of the placenta.

Atropine toxicity is characterized by dry mouth, burning sensation in the mouth, rapid pulse, mydriasis, blurred vision, photophobia, dry and flushed skin, restlessness, and excitement. **Fig. 4-8**

Physostigmine, given intravenously, counteracts both the peripheral and central side effects of atropine and other anticholinergic drugs, such as **thioridazine**

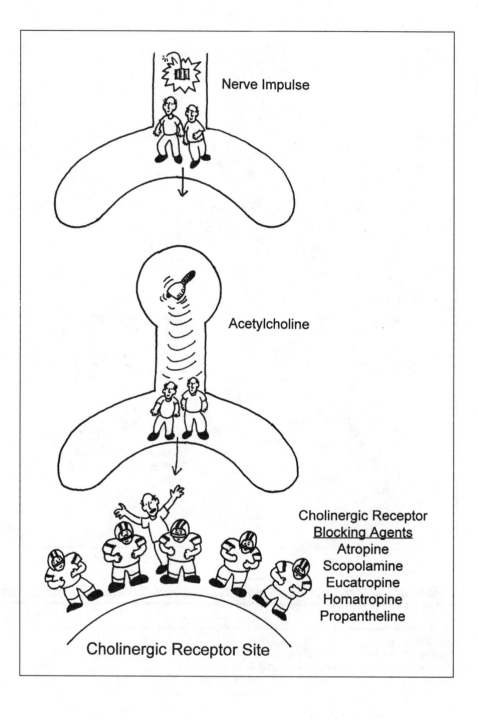

Nerve Impulse

Acetylcholine

Cholinergic Receptor
Blocking Agents
Atropine
Scopolamine
Eucatropine
Homatropine
Propantheline

Cholinergic Receptor Site

■ **Fig. 4-7** ■
Action of cholinergic receptor blocking agents.

(neuroleptic), **imipramine** (antidepressant), and **benztropine** (antiparkinsonian medication).

Methantheline and **propantheline** are synthetic derivatives that, beside their antimuscarinic effects, are ganglionic blocking agents and block the skeletal neuromuscular junction. Propantheline and **oxyphenonium** reduce gastric secretion, while **pirenzepine,** in addition to reducing gastric secretion, also reduces gastric motility.

Contraindication to Anticholinergic Agents

Conditions that are contraindications to the use of atropine and related drugs are glaucoma and prosta-

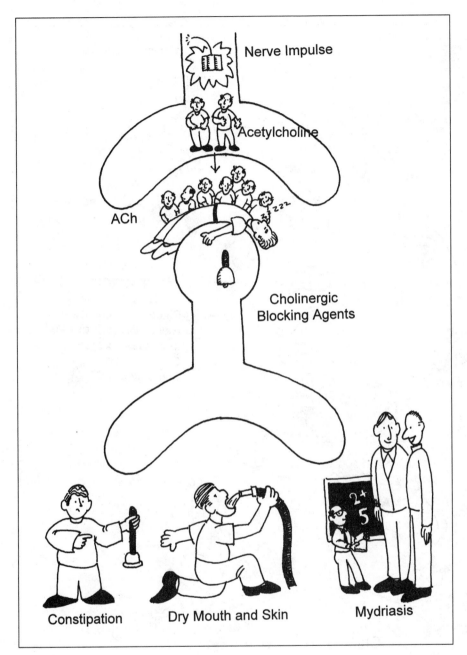

Nerve Impulse

Acetylcholine

ACh

Cholinergic
Blocking Agents

Constipation   Dry Mouth and Skin   Mydriasis

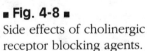

■ **Fig. 4-8** ■
Side effects of cholinergic
receptor blocking agents.

tic hypertrophy, in which they cause urinary retention.

Adrenergic Transmission

Neurochemical Basis of Adrenergic Transmission

Dopamine, norepinephrine, and epinephrine are classified as **catecholamines** and are synthesized according to the scheme depicted in ■ **Fig. 4-9** ■.

Tyrosine is converted to dopa by the rate-limiting enzyme **tyrosine hydroxylase,** which requires tetrahydrobiopterin, and is inhibited by alpha methyltyrosine. Dopa is decarboxylated to dopamine by **L-aromatic amino acid decarboxylase,** which requires pyridoxal phosphate (vitamin B_6) as a coenzyme. **Carbidopa,** which is used with levodopa in the treatment of parkinsonism, inhibits this enzyme. Dopamine is converted to norepinephrine by **dopamine beta-hydroxylase,** which requires ascorbic acid (vitamin C), and is

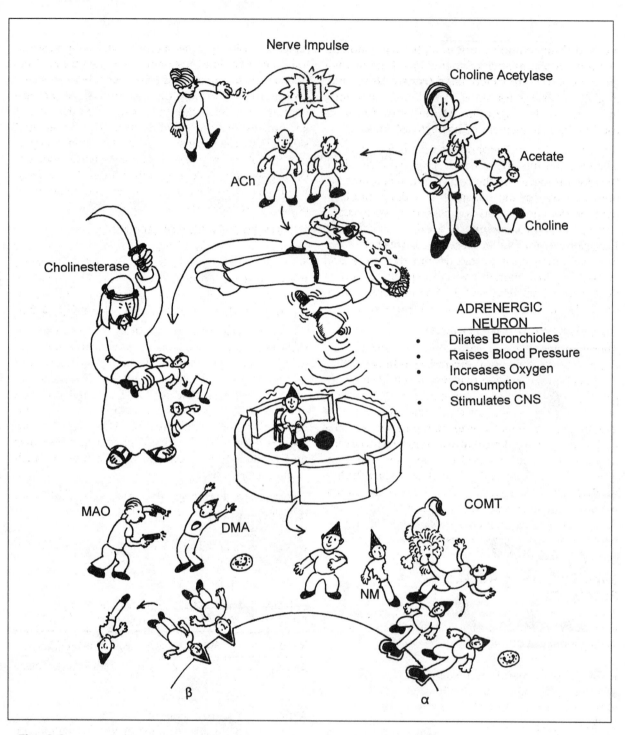

■ Fig. 4-9 ■
Synthesis, release, and actions of norepinephrine.

inhibited by diethyldithiocarbamate. Norepinephrine is converted to epinephrine by **phenylethanolamine-N-methyltransferase (PNMT),** requiring S-adenosylmethionine. The activity of PNMT is stimulated by **corticosteroids**.

The **catecholamine-synthesizing enzymes** are able to synthesize dopamine and norepinephrine not only from a physiologically occurring substrate such as levodopa but also from exogenous substrates such as **alpha methyldopa,** which is converted to alpha methyldopamine and in turn to alpha methylnorepinephrine. Alpha methyldopamine and alpha methylnorepinephrine are called **false transmitters,** and, in general (except for alpha methylnorepinephrine), they are weaker agonists. **Alpha-methyldopa** is used in the management of **hypertension**.

The action of norepinephrine is terminated by reuptake mechanisms, two of which have been identified. **Uptake 1** is located in the presynaptic membrane, requires energy for the transport, is sodium and temperature dependent, and is inhibited by **ouabain** (a cardiac glycoside), **cocaine** (a local anesthetic), and **imipramine** (an antidepressant). **Uptake 2** is located extraneuronally in various smooth muscles and glands, requires energy, and is temperature dependent. Approximately 20% of the amine is either taken up by the uptake 2 mechanism or is metabolized.

Catecholamine Metabolism

There are two enzymes capable of metabolizing catecholamines. The first is **monoamine oxidase** (MAO), a mitochondrial enzyme that oxidatively deaminates catecholamines, tyramine, serotonin, and histamine. MAO is further subclassified as either **monoamine oxidase A,** which metabolizes norepinephrine and is inhibited by **tranylcypromine,** and **monoamine oxidase B,** which metabolizes dopamine and is inhibited by **L-deprenyl** (selegiline). **Catechol-O-methyltransferase** (COMT), a soluble enzyme present mainly in the liver and kidney, is also found in postsynaptic neuronal elements. About 15% of norepinephrine is metabolized postsynaptically by COMT. See ■ **Fig. 4-9** ■

Classification of Adrenergic Receptors

Adrenergic receptors are classified as either alpha or beta receptors and are further subdivided into the following categories:

- Alpha$_1$: postsynaptic and excitatory
- Alpha$_2$: presynaptic and inhibitory
- Beta$_1$: postsynaptic and excitatory
- Beta$_2$: postsynaptic and inhibitory

The agonists and antagonists for these receptors are listed in ■ **Table 4-2** ■.

Salmeterol is a long-acting beta-adrenergic receptor agonist.

Denervation Supersensitivity

A denervated structure, whether it is a skeletal muscle or a postganglionic nerve fiber to an autonomic effector cell such as a smooth muscle, shows enhanced sensitivity to its agonists such as potassium ions, acetylcholine, histamine, and serotonin. This **denervation supersensitivity** becomes especially pronounced following the application of norepinephrine and is thought to be caused by the lack of an **amino uptake mechanism.** The innervated skeletal muscle is sensitive to acetylcholine only at the end plates, whereas the entire muscle fiber becomes sensitive following denervation. It is speculated that denervation results in the creation of additional receptor sites. See ■ **Fig. 4-9** ■

Adrenergic Receptor Agonists

Epinephrine acts on both alpha and beta receptors. **Norepinephrine** acts primarily on alpha receptors. **Isoproterenol** is a pure beta agonist. The functions associated with alpha receptors are vasoconstriction, mydriasis, and intestinal relaxation. See ■ **Fig. 4-9** ■

The functions associated with **beta receptors** are vasodilation, cardioacceleration, bronchial relaxation, positive inotropic effect, intestinal relaxation, and glycogenolysis and fatty acid release. The beta$_1$ receptors are responsible for cardiac stimulation and lipolysis. Beta$_2$ receptors are responsible for bronchodilation and vasodepression. Beta$_2$ agonists are especially useful in the treatment of asthma because they produce bronchodilation without causing much cardiac acceleration.

Therapeutic Applications - The therapeutic uses of epinephrine and its related drugs are:

- As a bronchodilator (beta$_2$ receptor activation in asthma)
- As a mydriatic (contracts radial muscle)

■ **Table 4-2** ■ Classification of Adrenergic Receptors, Agonists, and Antagonists

Receptors	Agonists	Antagonists
Alpha$_1$	Dopamine Epinephrine Norepinephrine	Prazosin Phenoxybenzamine Phentolamine
Alpha$_2$	Epinephrine Norepinephrine	Phenoxybenzamine Phentolamine
Beta$_1$	Dopamine Dobutamine Epinephrine Norepinephrine Isoproterenol	Propranolol Atenolol Metoprolol Esmolol Labetalol
Beta$_2$	Epinephrine Norepinephrine Isoproterenol	Propranolol Nadolol Labetalol Butoxamine

- In glaucoma (lowers intraocular pressure)
- For allergic reactions (prevents antigen-induced histamine releases)
- In hypotension (increases the mean pressure)
- As a nasal decongestant (**mephentermine**)
- As a local anesthesia (produces a bloodless field of operation, delays absorption and yields a longer duration of anesthetic action, and protects the brain and heart against the toxic effects of local anesthetics)
- As cardiac stimulants (epinephrine or isoproterenol may be injected in heart block to improve atrioventricular conduction velocity and stimulate ventricular automaticity)

Pharmacology of Other Adrenergic (Sympathomimetics) Receptor Stimulants -

In general, these sympathomimetic agents can be divided into three categories: **direct-acting agents,** which exert their effect directly on the receptor sites; **indirect-acting agents** such as amphetamine and tyamine, which exert their effects by releasing norepinephrine; and **mixed-acting agents** such as ephedrine and to a certain extent amphetamine, which are direct agonists and also release norepinephrine.

Sympathomimetic agents are contraindicated in patients with hypertension and hyperthyroidism. In addition, they should not be used in combination with anesthetics that sensitize the heart to the effects of catecholamine.

Adrenergic Blocking Drugs

These adrenergic blocking (antiadrenergic) agents exert their effects by blocking the access of circulating epinephrine, norepinephrine, and other sympathomimetic amines to the adrenergic receptors.

Alpha-Adrenergic Blockers

Phenoxybenzamine (Dibenzyline) is a noncompetitive alpha-adrenergic receptor blocker, and its action cannot be nullified by increasing the amount of agonist or agonists. It causes **epinephrine reversal** in that the administration of epinephrine after pretreatment with phenoxybenzamine elicits vasodilation, and, conversely, phenoxybenzamine reverses epinephrine-mediated vasoconstriction to vasodilation.

Phentolamine (Regitine) is a competitive alpha-adrenergic blocker, and its action can be nullified by increasing the amount of agonist or agonists. Phenoxybenzamine and phentolamine have limited therapeutic usefulness. They are occasionally used in the treatment of peripheral vascular disease (**Raynaud disease**), in the diagnosis of **pheochromocytoma,** and during surgery for pheochromocytoma.

Prazosin (Minipress), which is used to treat **hypertension,** causes alpha-adrenergic blockade and direct vasodilation.

Beta-Adrenergic Blockers

These beta-adrenergic blockers are competitive blockers of both $beta_1$ and $beta_2$ receptor sites. These agents block sympathomimetic actions other than vasoconstriction, including vasodilatation, cardiac acceleration, increased cardiac output, bronchiolar dilatation, and hyperglycemia. They are used therapeutically for cardiac arrhythmias, digitalis-induced arrhythmias, ventricular tachycardia, atrial flutter or fibrillation, pheochromocytoma, anginal pain, hypertension, and thyrotoxicosis.

The **pharmacologic characteristics of various beta-blocking agents** are summarized in ■ **Table 4-3** ■.

Beta-adrenergic blocking agents that are **cardioselective** are acebutolol, atenolol, and metoprolol. Beta-adrenergic blocking agents that are **not cardioselective** are alprenolol, nadolol, oxprenolol, pindolol, propranolol, sotalol, and timolol.

■ **Table 4-3** ■ The Pharmacologic Characteristics of Beta-Adrenergic Receptor Blocking Agents

Drug Name	ISA	$Beta_1$ Selectivity	Alpha-Blocking Activity
Propranolol	−	−	−
Timolol	−	−	−
Metoprolol	−	+	−
Nadolol	−	−	−
Atenolol	−	+	−
Acebutolol	+−	+	−
Labetaolol	−	−	+
Pindolol	+++	−	−
Penbutolol	+−	−	−

ISA = intrinsic sympathomimetic activity; + = the drug possesses the assigned property; − = the drug does not possess the assigned property.

III

Neuropharmacology

CHAPTER 5

Drugs for Parkinson's Disease

Four separate groups of symptoms constitute the symptom complex that makes up parkinsonism: tremor, akinesia or bradykinesia, rigidity, and loss of postural reflexes.

Synthesis of Dopamine

Tyrosine is converted to dopa by a rate-limiting enzyme, **tyrosine hydroxylase,** which requires tetrahydrobiopterin, and is inhibited by alpha-methyltyrosine. Dopa is decarboxylated to dopamine by **L-aromatic amino acid decarboxylase,** which requires pyridoxal phosphate (vitamin B_6) as a co-enzyme. **Carbidopa,** which is used with **levodopa** in the treatment of parkinsonism, inhibits this enzyme. Dopamine is metabolized by **monoamine oxidase B**, and this enzyme is inhibited by **selegiline.** ■ Fig. 5-1 ■

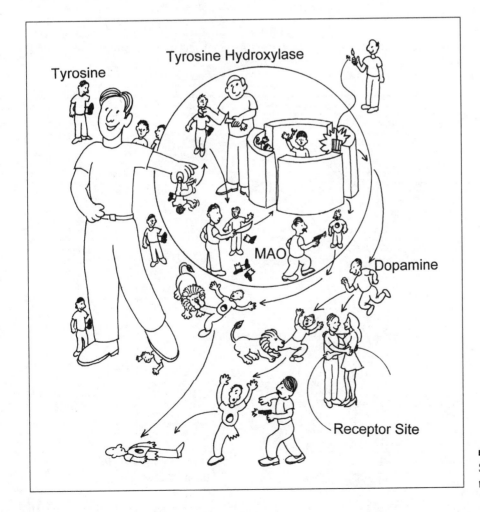

■ Fig. 5-1 ■
Synthesis, release, and action of dopamine.

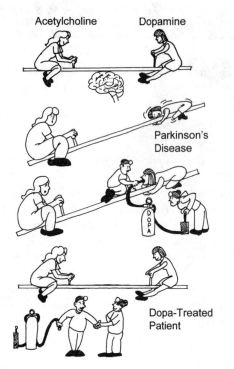

Acetylcholine   Dopamine

Parkinson's
Disease

Dopa-Treated
Patient

■ Fig. 5-2 ■
Parkinson's disease is a striatal dopamine deficiency
syndrome and is treated with levodopa.

Actions of Acetylcholine and Dopamine

Neurochemically, Parkinson's syndrome is considered
a **striatal dopamine-deficiency syndrome,** and the
main **extrapyramidal symptoms** — tremor, akinesia,
and rigidity — correlate positively with the degree of
this deficiency. Although eight separate neurotransmitters interact in the nigro-striato-nigral loop, the basic
therapeutic problem in parkinsonism has been to find
suitable compounds that (1) increase the concentration
of dopamine by levodopa, **■ Fig. 5-2 ■** (2) stimulate
the dopamine receptor sites directly by bromocriptine,
or (3) suppress the activity at cholinergic receptor
sites. **■ Fig. 5-3 ■** Therefore, drugs fall into two main
categories: those that increase dopaminergic function
and those that inhibit cholinergic hyperactivity.

Agents That Increase Dopaminergic Functions

Several mechanisms may enhance the activity at
dopamine receptor sites in the striatum:

- Increasing the synthesis of dopamine (**levodopa**)
- Inhibiting the catabolism of dopamine (L-deprenyl)
  (**selegiline**)

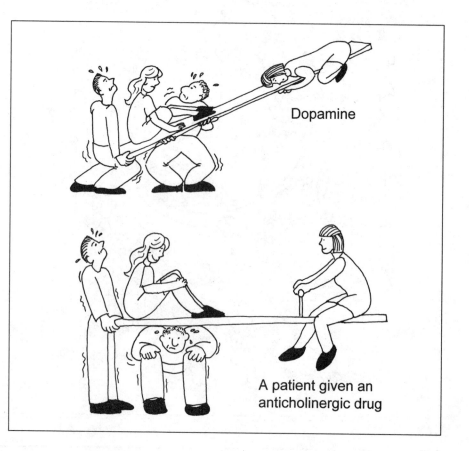

Dopamine

A patient given an
anticholinergic drug

■ Fig. 5-3 ■
Parkinson's disease causes
cholinergic hyperactivity
and may be treated with
anticholinergic agents.

- Stimulating the dopamine receptor sites directly (**bromocriptine** and **pergolide**)
- Blocking the uptake and enhancing the release of dopamine (**amantadine**)

Of these possibilities, the most effective means of treating parkinsonism has been to enhance the synthesis of dopamine.

Levodopa

Current practice is to give levodopa in combination with **carbidopa,** a peripheral dopa-decarboxylase inhibitor.

The first signs of improvement are usually a subjective feeling of well-being accompanied by increased vigor. The symptoms yield in the following sequence: first the akinesia, then the rigidity, and finally the tremor, which disappears slowly and incompletely. If the drug is stopped, the symptoms reappear in the reverse order: tremor, rigidity, and then akinesia. The postural abnormality responds less effectively to medications. ■ **Fig. 5-4** ■

Emetic Action of Levodopa - Enhancing the dose of carbidopa attenuates the emetic actions of levodopa. The use of a phenothiazine antiemetic (such as **chlorpromazine**, which blocks dopamine receptor sites in the brain and therefore counteracts the beneficial effects of levodopa) is discouraged. ■ **Fig. 5-5** ■

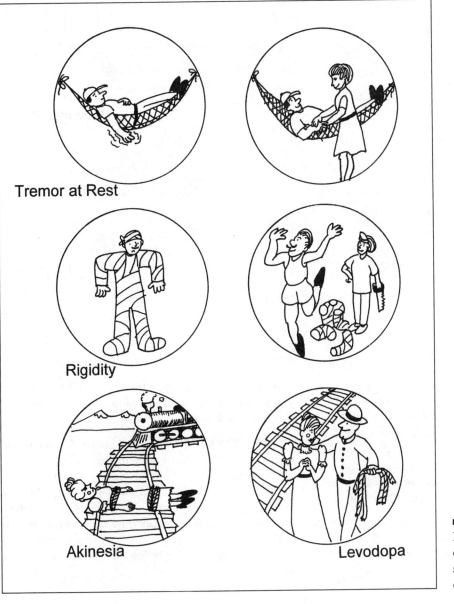

Tremor at Rest

Rigidity

Akinesia

Levodopa

■ **Fig. 5-4** ■
Beneficial effects of levodopa in alleviating the symptoms of Parkinson's disease.

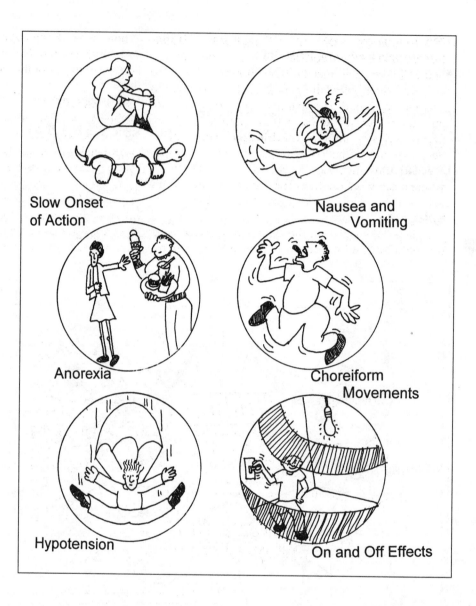

Slow Onset of Action

Nausea and Vomiting

Anorexia

Choreiform Movements

Hypotension

On and Off Effects

■ **Fig. 5-5** ■
Side effects of levodopa.

Involuntary Movements - The development of involuntary movements may limit the usefulness of levodopa. This **peak dose dyskinesia** is usually manifested in the form of choreic movements that involve the hands, arms, legs, and face. To avoid these involuntary movements, the frequency of drug administration must usually be increased and the individual dose of levodopa decreased. See ■ **Fig. 5-5** ■

Cardiovascular Disorders - Therapeutic doses of levodopa produce hypotension and cardiac stimulation by activating the beta₁ receptor site in the heart. In some elderly patients, it may produce cardiac ar-rhythmias. The cardiac stimulation is blocked by **propranolol,** the beta-adrenergic receptor-blocking agent, or **carbidopa**.

On-Off Phenomenon - The **on-off phenomenon** is a sudden loss of effectiveness with the abrupt onset of **akinesia** — "off" effects — that may last for minutes or hours. This is followed by an equally sudden return of effectiveness — "on" effects — which may be even be accompanied by **hyperkinesia**. The effect is so sudden that it has been compared to the action of a light switch being turned on and off. See ■ **Fig. 5-5** ■

Pharmacology of a Peripheral Dopa-Decarboxylase Inhibitor - When administered orally, levodopa is metabolized substantially in the gut and tissues; very little penetrates into the brain to become converted to dopamine. The combined administration of levodopa with a peripheral dopa-decarboxylase inhibitor (**carbidopa**) substantially decreases the formation of dopamine in the periphery and thus increases its formation in the brain, where it can work on the corpus striatum. ■ **Fig. 5-6** ■

Selegiline

Selegiline is effective in the treatment of parkinsonism because it inhibits the catabolism of dopamine.

There are indications that selegiline alone can slow the progression of Parkinson's disease, when taken in the early stages of the disease.

Bromocriptine

As parkinsonism progresses, the activity of dopa-decarboxylase may become so reduced that it cannot adequately decarboxylate dopa to dopamine. In this case, it may be possible to stimulate the dopamine receptor sites located postsynaptically using compounds such as bromocriptine or pergolide. ■ **Fig. 5-7** ■ Bromocriptine has a longer duration of action than levodopa and is particularly useful in patients suffering from a high incidence of on-off phenomenon.

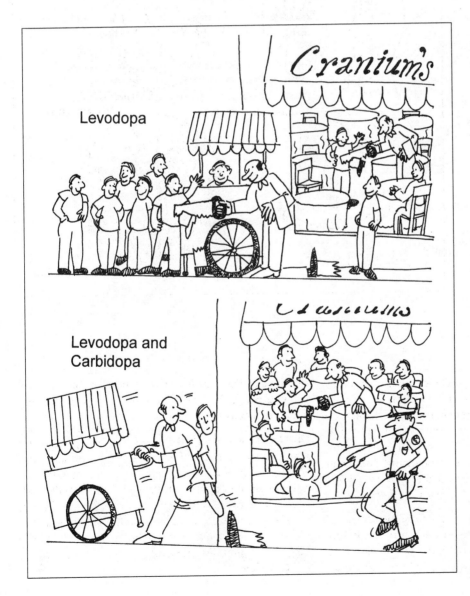

■ **Fig. 5-6** ■
The action of carbidopa, a peripheral dopa-decarboxylase inhibitor.

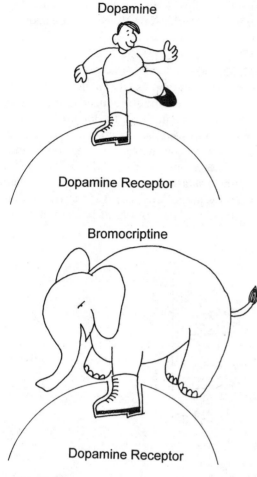

Dopamine

Dopamine Receptor

Bromocriptine

Dopamine Receptor

■ **Fig. 5-7** ■

Bromocriptine is an agonist at the dopamine receptors.

Amantadine

Although the actions of amantadine are still not fully understood, there is some evidence that the drug inhibits the uptake of dopamine into the synaptosomes. In addition, amantadine has an indirect **amphetamine**-like effect in that it releases dopamine.

Agents That Inhibit Cholinergic Hyperactivity

In parkinsonian patients, the deficiency of dopamine causes the cholinergic receptors to be hyperactive. See ■ **Fig. 5-3** ■ Therefore, **anticholinergic drugs** may be used to mitigate some of the symptoms. These agents include **trihexyphenidyl** (Artane) and **benztropine** (Cogentin).

Contraindications to the use of anticholinergic drugs in treating parkinsonism are the same as those for atropine: glaucoma, prostatic hypertrophy, myasthenia gravis, stenosing peptic ulcer, and duodenal or pyloric obstruction. **Urinary retention** and **tachycardia** should be heeded and regarded as signs of impending toxicity.

CHAPTER 6

Anticonvulsants

Therapeutic Objectives

The main therapeutic objective in the pharmacologic management of epilepsy is the complete suppression of all seizures without impairing CNS functions. Successful drug therapy also depends on the administration of agents that are appropriate for the patient's seizure type. Agents must be given in doses that are sufficient to control the seizures without causing troublesome adverse effects.

Basic Mechanism of Epilepsy

The basic mechanisms underlying convulsive disorders are so diverse that to seek a single cause would be a gross oversimplification. Rather, a number of different disorders, singly or in combination, may result in seizure discharge. However, one of the better-characterized defects concerns **gamma-aminobutyric acid** (GABA) and its role as a neurotransmitter. Biochemical lesions that interrupt the synthesis, storage, release, or postsynaptic actions of inhibitory neurotransmitters such as GABA lead to disinhibition of neurons.

The synthesis of GABA is achieved by decarboxylation of glutamate, which is mediated by glutamic acid decarboxylase (GAD), a rate-limiting enzyme. Several compounds that have been found to lower the threshold for seizures or frankly elicit seizures have also been found to inhibit GAD. Hence, reducing available GABA levels appears to represent a possible epileptogenic mechanism.

Several agents related to GABA metabolism and its receptors have been found to possess some degree of antiepileptic activity. Specific **benzodiazepine** and **barbiturate** receptors have been identified in the postsynaptic membrane, which, when activated by a benzodiazepine or barbiturate, enhance GABA binding to postsynaptic GABA receptors, resulting in prolonged chloride conductance and increased inhibition. ■ **Fig. 6-1** ■

Drugs Effective in Tonic-Clonic Seizures (Grand Mal) and Complex Partial Seizures

Hydantoin Derivatives

The hydantoin derivatives are **phenytoin** (diphenylhydantoin) and **mephenytoin** (Mesantoin).

Phenytoin

PHARMACOKINETICS - On passage into the small intestine, where the pH is basic (7.0–7.5), phenytoin exists in a **nonionized form** that favors its absorption. Absorption is highest from the duodenum and decreases rapidly in the lower parts of the small intestine.

After absorption, as much as 92–93% of phenytoin becomes bound to plasma proteins, allowing only 7–8% of the drug to remain free. Circumstances or drugs that alter the extent of protein binding will significantly affect phenytoin's therapeutic usefulness and may also precipitate phenytoin toxicity.

Phenytoin becomes metabolized in the liver to **hydroxyphenytoin,** which is an inactive metabolite. Hydroxyphenytoin is then conjugated with glucuronic acid and excreted by the kidneys.

PHARMACODYNAMICS - Phenytoin limits the development of maximal seizure activity and reduces the spread of the seizure process from an epileptic focus. It is a nonsedating anticonvulsant. ■ **Fig. 6-2** ■

Phenytoin reduces calcium transport at the outer nerve membrane by blocking its high-affinity binding sites. This reduces the release of norepinephrine, which is necessary for the generation of posttetanic potentiation, and the spread of the impending seizure process is curtailed. ■ **Fig. 6-3** ■

Phenytoin decreases the inward sodium current. Furthermore, when the intracellular concentration of sodium is elevated, phenytoin is thought to stimulate **Na$^+$K$^+$ ATPase** to reestablish the ionic gradient.

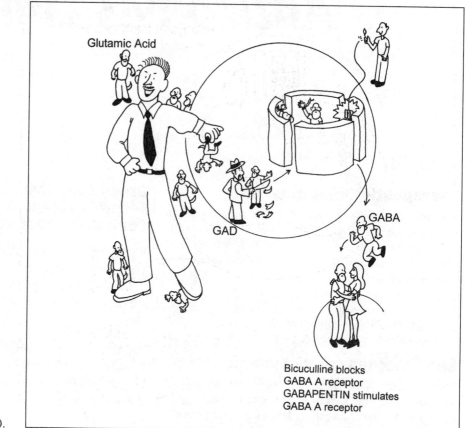

■Fig. 6-1 ■
Synthesis, release, and action of gamma-aminobutyric acid (GABA).

Bicuculline blocks
GABA A receptor
GABAPENTIN stimulates
GABA A receptor

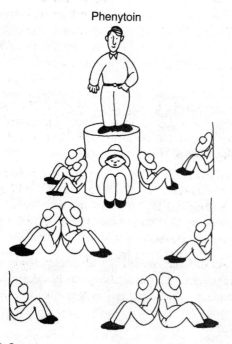

■Fig. 6-2 ■
Among antiepileptic agents, phenytoin causes no sedation.

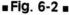

■ Fig. 6-4 ■ The activity of Na⁺K⁺ ATPase is reduced in the brains of epileptic patients.

A third concept is that phenytoin enhances GABA-ergic transmission.

SIDE EFFECTS AND TOXICITY - Phenytoin may cause **nystagmus, diplopia, staggering,** and **ataxia.** These side effects are generally regarded as dose-dependent.
■ Fig. 6-5 ■ Phenytoin causes **gingival hyperplasia.** Other medications causing gingival hyperplasia are **cyclosporine, nifedipine, diltiazem, verapamil,** and **nitrendipine.**

Phenytoin causes **hypertrichosis** in 5% of patients; it occurs several months after the initiation of therapy and is either slowly reversible or irreversible.

INDICATIONS - Phenytoin has been approved for the management of **tonic-clonic seizures** (grand mal) and **complex partial seizures**.

Mephenytoin - Mephenytoin is used for the treatment of tonic-clonic, simple partial, and complex partial seizures in patients who have become refractory to phenytoin or other drugs. The incidence of severe or fatal hypersensitivity reactions is far higher than

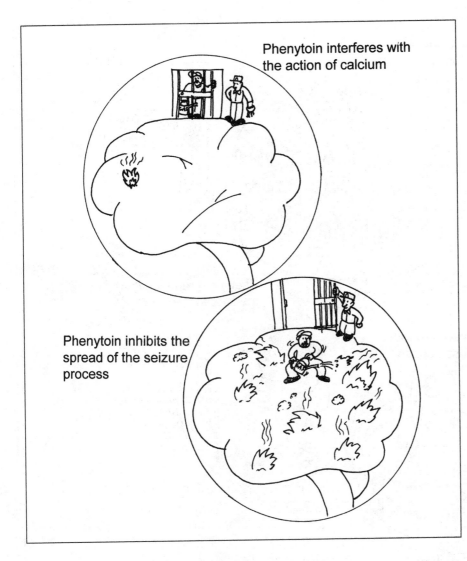

Phenytoin interferes with the action of calcium

Phenytoin inhibits the spread of the seizure process

■**Fig. 6-3** ■
Phenytoin, by competing with the action of calcium, prevents the spread of seizure activity.

that reported for phenytoin. Therefore, it should not be used with other agents such as **trimethadione**, that may cause similar effects. ■ **Fig. 6-6** ■

Barbiturate Derivatives

The barbiturate derivatives are **mephobarbital** (Mebaral), **phenobarbital** (Luminal), and **metharbital** (Gemonil) and the related anticonvulsant **primidone** (Mysoline).

In the body, mephobarbital is demethylated to phenobarbital. Therefore, the antiepileptic effects of mephobarbital may be due in part to phenobarbital. ■ **Fig. 6-7** ■

Phenobarbital

PHARMACOKINETICS - Phenobarbital is absorbed from the small intestine. As much as 50% binds to albumin, and it is metabolized in the liver to **hydroxy-**

phenobarbital. Approximately 20–25% of phenobarbital is excreted in the urine unchanged. It has a very long elimination half-life — up to 140 hours. ■ **Fig. 6-8** ■

Phenobarbital induces hepatic microsomal drug-metabolizing enzymes. The sudden withdrawal of phenobarbital may precipitate withdrawal seizures. Therefore, the doses should be tapered gradually whenever discontinuation is contemplated.

PHARMACODYNAMICS - Phenobarbital inhibits post-tetanic potentiation and especially raises the seizure threshold. Phenobarbital is thought to enhance the presynaptic release of GABA and simultaneously reduce the postsynaptic uptake of GABA.

SIDE EFFECTS AND TOXICITY - Compared to phenytoin, phenobarbital is a relatively safe compound. Rarely, a morbilliform rash occurs. In some

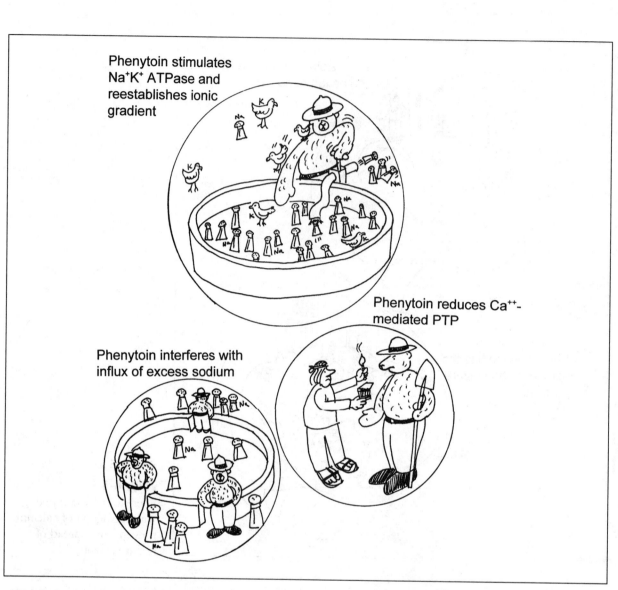

■ Fig. 6-4 ■

Phenytoin reduces the influx of Na⁺ and by stimulating the activity of Na⁺K⁺ ATPase reestablishes ionic gradient in the epileptic neurons.

patients, however, heavy sedation, reduction in activity, and impairment in cognition may be pronounced.

INDICATIONS - Phenobarbital has a broad spectrum of antiepileptic activity and efficacy. It is often used by itself or in combination with phenytoin. **■ Fig. 6-9 ■**

Primidone - Primidone is indicated in the treatment of tonic-clonic and partial seizures. Since the administration of primidone essentially yields three anticonvulsants in the body, it may be superior to phenobarbital for some patients. See **■ Fig. 6-7 ■**

Mephobarbital - Mephobarbital causes less sedation and hypersensitivity reactions than phenobarbital.

Iminostilbene Derivatives

Carbamazepine and Oxcarbazepine - After absorption, carbamazepine is bound to plasma proteins to the extent of 60–70%. Carbamazepine is metabolized to 10,11-epoxide and 10,11-dihydroxide derivatives of carbamazepine, some of which are excreted unchanged; the other portion is conjugated with glucuronic acid. The 10,11-epoxide derivatives are active anticonvulsants.

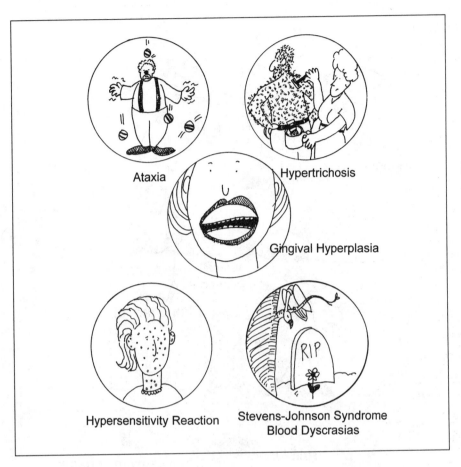

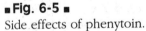

Ataxia

Hypertrichosis

Gingival Hyperplasia

Hypersensitivity Reaction

Stevens-Johnson Syndrome
Blood Dyscrasias

■Fig. 6-5 ■
Side effects of phenytoin.

The mode and mechanism of carbamazepine action are similar but not identical to those of phenytoin. ■ **Fig. 6-10** ■ In high but therapeutic doses, carbamazepine decreases sodium and potassium conductances and increases the **taurine** level, decreases the glutamic acid concentration, and enhances GABAergic transmission.

INDICATIONS - Carbamazepine is as effective as phenobarbital, phenytoin, and primidone in the prevention of **generalized tonic-clonic seizures** but is significantly more effective than the others in the treatment of **complex partial seizures.** Carbamazepine is also used for the management of **trigeminal neuralgia** and **complex partial seizures with temporal lobe symptomatology.** Besides its antiepileptic effect, carbamazepine possesses sedative, anticholinergic, antidepressant, muscle relaxant, antiarrhythmic, antidiuretic, and neuromuscular transmission inhibitory actions. Therefore, carbamazepine has been used in the treatment of childhood episodic behavior disorder, multiple sclerosis, central diabetes insipidus, and dystonia. Additional clinical trials should clarify the usefulness of carbamazepine in these conditions.

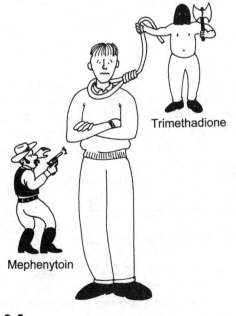

Trimethadione

Mephenytoin

■Fig. 6-6 ■
Mephenytoin and trimethadione produce high incidences of hypersensitivity reactions and should not be used together.

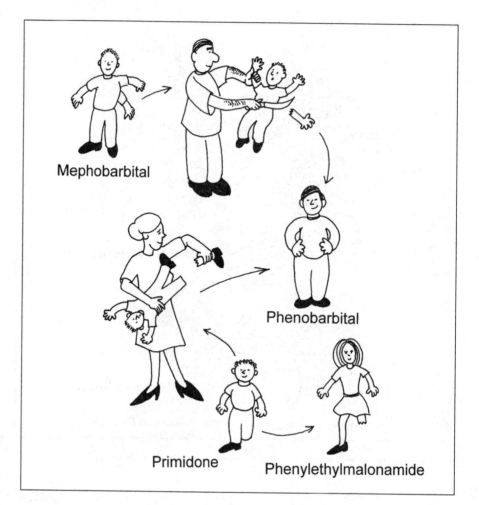

■ Fig. 6-7 ■
Primidone and mephobarbital become converted to phenobarbital.

Mephobarbital

Phenobarbital

Primidone

Phenylethylmalonamide

Drugs Effective in Absence (Petit Mal) Seizures

Succinamide Derivatives

The succinamide derivatives are **ethosuximide** (Zarontin), **methsuximide** (Celontin), and **phensuximide** (Milontin).

Ethosuximide is more effective than methsuximide and phensuximide. It does not bind to plasma proteins. It appears in the spinal fluid 30–60 minutes after administration and crosses the placental barrier. Ethosuximide is metabolized primarily by hydroxylation, and the metabolite is not an active anticonvulsant. The only indication for ethosuximide is the treatment of absence seizures.

Oxazolidine Derivatives

The oxazolidine derivatives are **trimethadione** (Tridione) and **paramethadione** (Paradione).

The consequences of trimethadione **toxicity** consist of hematologic side effects (neutropenia, pancytopenia), hemeralopia (day blindness), photophobia, diplopia, dermatologic side effects (rash and erythema multiforme), CNS side effects (drowsiness and tolerance), nephrotoxic syndrome (albuminuria), and teratogenic effects such as **fetal trimethadione syndrome.** Trimethadione is indicated only for the control of absence seizures that are not responsive or have become refractory to treatment with less toxic substances such as ethosuximide or valproic acid.

Propylpentanoic Acid Derivatives

The chief propylpentanoic acid derivative used in the treatment of absence seizures is **valproic acid.** Valproic acid (Depakene) is absorbed rapidly, and from 85–90% binds to plasma proteins. It is able to displace bound phenytoin or phenobarbital and is metabolized to metabolites, notably 2-propyl-2-pentenoic acid and

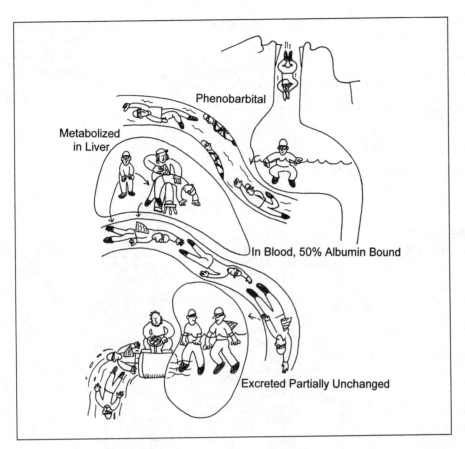

■Fig. 6-8 ■
Pharmacokinetic properties
of phenobarbital.

Phenobarbital

Metabolized
in Liver

In Blood, 50% Albumin Bound

Excreted Partially Unchanged

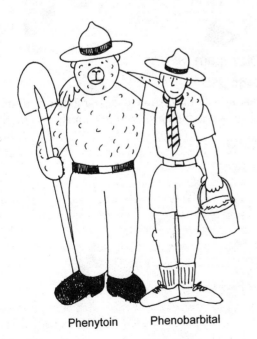

Phenytoin   Phenobarbital

■Fig. 6-9 ■
Phenytoin and phenobarbital are often used
together in grand mal epilepsy.

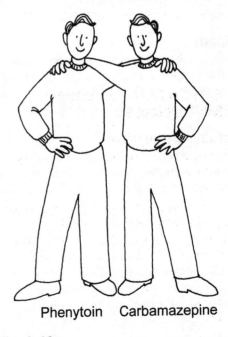

Phenytoin   Carbamazepine

■Fig. 6-10 ■
The mechanisms of antiepileptic actions of phenytoin and carbamazepine are similar.

2-propyl-4-pentenoic acid, that are anticonvulsants. Valproic acid has a short half-life of 8–9 hours.

The mechanism of action of valproic acid has been postulated to be its enhancement of GABAergic transmission.

Valproic acid has a broad spectrum of anticonvulsant activity and is effective in the control of absence seizures, with an effectiveness equivalent to that of ethosuximide. It is also effective in the treatment of myoclonic and tonic-clonic seizures, especially those occurring concomitantly with absence seizures.

Drugs Effective in Seizure Disorders Including Status Epilepticus

The benzodiazepine derivatives are **diazepam** (Valium), **chlorazepate** (Tranxene), and **clonazepam** (Clonopin). Both diazepam and clonazepam interact with the benzodiazepine receptor sites, which in turn enhances the postsynaptic GABAergic transmission. ■ **Fig. 6-11** ■

Diazepam

The IV administration of diazepam produces transient high serum and brain concentrations of the agent, which is effective in aborting persistent and uninterrupted tonic-clonic convulsions. The metabolites of diazepam, **desmethyldiazepam** and **oxazepam,** are active anticonvulsants.

Clonazepam

Clonazepam is a **broad-spectrum anticonvulsant.** It may be used by itself or in combination with other antiepileptic drugs for the control of absence seizures (typical and atypical petit mal), infantile spasms (in-fantile myoclonic and massive spasms), myoclonic seizures, and atonic seizures (akinetic). In addition, it is believed to be effective in the treatment of tonic-clonic (grand mal) and complex partial (psychomotor-temporal lobe) seizures.

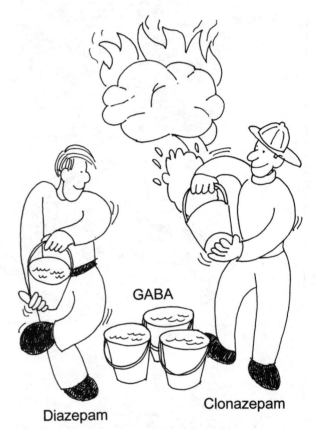

■**Fig. 6-11** ■
Diazepam and clonazepam exert their anticonvulsant properties by enhancing GABAergic transmission.

IV

Psychopharmacology

CHAPTER 7

The Neuroleptics and Schizophrenia

Symptoms of Schizophrenia

Type I schizophrenia is characterized by acute psychosis with positive symptoms, absence of intellectual impairment, and a good response to neuroleptic drugs. **Type II** schizophrenia is associated with chronic schizophrenia, intellectual impairment, cerebroventricular enlargement, negative symptoms, and a poor response to neuroleptics.

Dopamine, Schizophrenia, and the Neuroleptics

Although an alteration in the levels of acetylcholine, norepinephrine, and serotonin plus an imbalance between the concentrations of gamma-aminobutyric acid (GABA) and glutamic acid have been implicated as etiologic factors in both schizophrenia and depression, **dopamine receptors** may play a role in the etiology of schizophrenia and in the mechanism of action and side effects of neuroleptics. Dopaminergic hyperactivity in the mesocortical and mesolimbic systems has been thought to contribute to schizophrenic symptomatology.

Amphetamine (which causes the release of dopamine) and **levodopa** (which brings about an increase in the dopamine level) aggravate schizophrenia. Compounds that block dopamine receptors in the **mesocortical** and **mesolimbic systems** (chlorpromazine and haloperidol) are **antipsychotic.** The more potent a compound is in blocking dopamine receptors (e.g., haloperidol), the more potent it is as a **neuroleptic.** Compounds that do not block dopamine receptor sites (e.g., promethazine) are devoid of antipsychotic activity. Classic neuroleptics such as chlorpromazine block dopamine$_1$ (D$_1$) and dopamine$_2$ (D$_2$) receptor sites, whereas atypical neuroleptics such as clozapine block D$_2$ receptors only. Clozapine causes negligible or no extrapyramidal side effects. ■ **Figs. 7-1 through 7-4** ■

The Neuroleptics

Phenothiazine Derivatives

These agents differ in their potency but not their efficacy. Long-acting injectable drugs such as **fluphenazine decanoate** and **fluphenazine enanthate,** which need to be given only once every 2 or 3 weeks, are increasingly used in outpatients and in patients who are uncooperative and noncompliant. Phenothiazine derivatives devoid of neuroleptic activity also exist. **Promethazine** (Phenergan) is an **antihistaminic; ethopropazine** (Parsidol) has a **muscle relaxant** effect (because of its anticholinergic action, it may be used in **parkinsonism** as well).

In discussing the neuroleptics, the pharmacology of **chlorpromazine** is discussed as a prototype drug, and all other drugs compared with it.

Pharmacokinetics - Chlorpromazine is well absorbed mainly from the jejunum. It is extensively metabolized in the liver, which produces several active metabolites. When given intramuscularly, the phenothiazine neuroleptics avoid metabolic degradation (first-pass metabolism), making them more beneficial as long-acting depot antipsychotics.

Central Nervous System Effects - Chlorpromazine produces a **tranquility** that is characterized by a detached serenity without depression of mental faculties or clouding of consciousness.

In general, chlorpromazine and other neuroleptics **reduce spontaneous motor activity** in proportion to their dosages. Chlorpromazine depresses conditioned avoidance behavior but not escape behavior. Phenothiazine derivatives reduce the **seizure threshold.**

Antiemetic Effect - The nausea and vomiting associated with circulating physical agents (radiation therapy and virus particles) and chemical agents

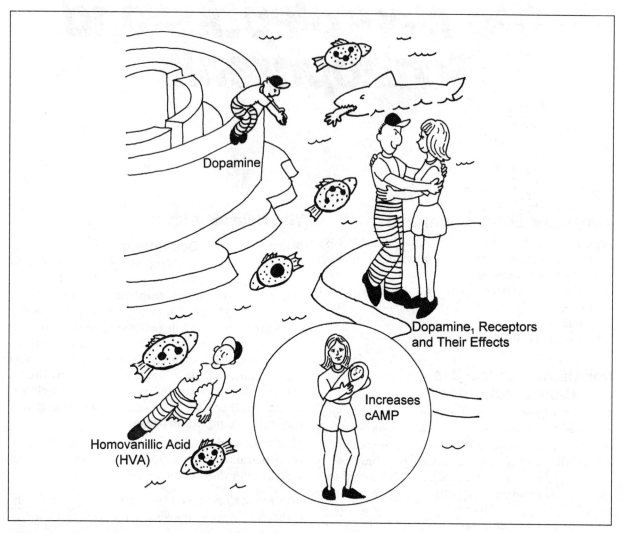

■ Fig. 7-1 ■
Interaction of dopamine with dopamine receptors.

(toxins and cancer chemotherapeutic agents) that stimulate the **chemoreceptor trigger zone for emesis** are treated with prochlorperazine or promethazine. **■ Fig. 7-5 ■**

Hypothermic Effects - The phenothiazine derivatives are hypothermic, with the extent of hypothermia depending on the dosage and the environmental temperature. See **■ Fig. 7-5 ■**

Antiadrenergic and Hypotensive Effects - Phenothiazine derivatives cause postural or orthostatic hypotension. The hypotension is due to direct vasodilation and an alpha-adrenergic receptor-blocking effect. See **■ Fig. 7-5 ■**

Hepatotoxicity - Phenothiazine derivatives have been observed to cause jaundice in 5% of patients. The jaundice is accompanied by intense pruritus, fever, chills, nausea, epigastric or right upper quadrant abdominal pain, and malaise. The jaundice is not dose dependent and develops after a typical delay of 2–3 weeks. With discontinuation of medication, the prognosis has been excellent. See **■ Fig. 7-5 ■**

Endocrine Effects - Phenothiazine derivatives cause reversible **galactorrhea** and **gynecomastia**. See **■ Fig. 7-5 ■** Thioridazine causes a reversible ejaculation disorder, in that erection and orgasm occur without ejaculation. Chlorpromazine, by preventing the

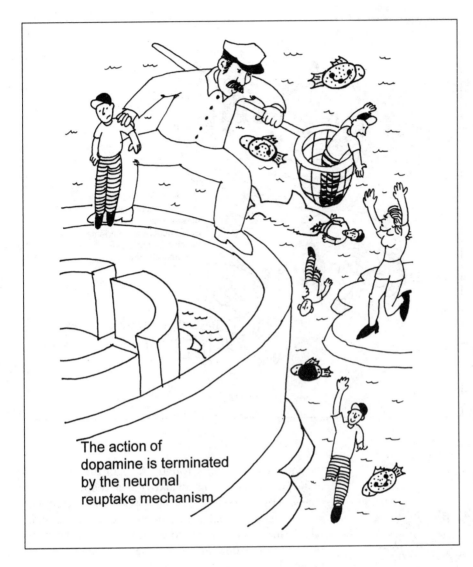

The action of dopamine is terminated by the neuronal reuptake mechanism

■ **Fig. 7-2** ■
Dopamine is either catabolized or its action is terminated by the amine uptake mechanism.

release of insulin, may cause diabetes mellitus in a borderline individual or destabilize a diabetic patient. ■ **Fig. 7-5** ■

Hematologic Effects - Chlorpromazine causes agranulocytosis. See ■ **Fig. 7-5** ■

Dermatologic Effects - **Solar sensitivity,** which occurs only in sun-exposed areas of the body such as the hands and face, can be prevented by having patients avoid exposure to the sun. See ■ **Fig. 7-5** ■

Allergic dermatitis, which may be maculopapular, urticarial, or pruritic, should be regarded as a hypersensitivity reaction. Medication should be discontinued and other supportive therapy initiated.

Pigment retinopathy is manifested by the deposition of dotlike particles in the anterior capsular and subcapsular portion of the lens, pupillary area, cornea, conjunctiva, and retina.

Extrapyramidal Side Effects - **Akathisia** is characterized by an inability to sit still, by shifting of the legs and tapping of feet while sitting, and by rocking and shifting of the weight while standing. Reducing the total dosage of neuroleptic medications and the addition of an **anticholinergic drug**, one of the **benzodiazepine** derivatives, or **propranolol** have been shown to reduce the severity of akathisia. See ■ **Fig. 7-5** ■

Dystonia is characterized by an exaggerated posturing of the head, neck, or jaw; by spastic contraction of

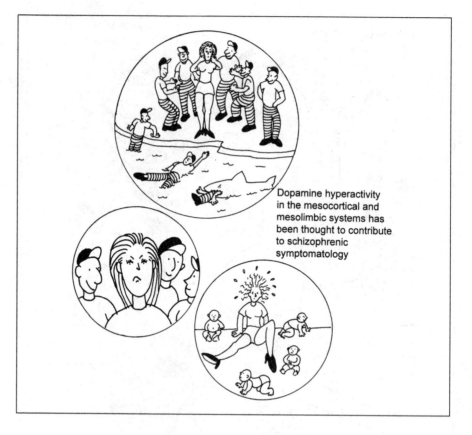

■Fig. 7-3 ■
Dopaminergic receptors play a role in both the etiology of schizophrenia and the mechanism of actions and side effects of neuroleptics.

Dopamine hyperactivity in the mesocortical and mesolimbic systems has been thought to contribute to schizophrenic symptomatology

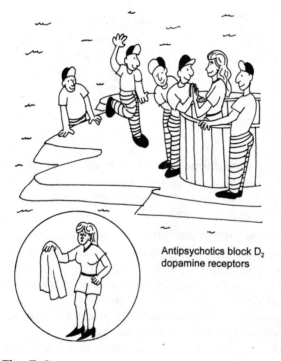

Antipsychotics block D_2 dopamine receptors

■Fig. 7-4 ■
The more potent a compound is in blocking dopamine receptors, the more potent it is as an antipsychotic.

the muscles of the lips, tongue, face, or throat, which makes drinking, eating, swallowing, and speech difficult; and by torticollis, retrocollis, opisthotonus, distress, and ultimately anoxia. Neuroleptic-induced dystonia, which may occur in children treated actively with phenothiazine derivatives for their antiemetic properties, disappears in sleep and is treated effectively with **diphenhydramine hydrochloride** (Benadryl), which possesses both anticholinergic and antihistaminic properties.

Parkinsonian - These symptoms, which are due to blockade of dopaminergic receptor sites in the striatum, are lessened by reducing the dosage of neuroleptics and by the oral administration of anticholinergic compounds, such as **trihexyphenidyl hydrochloride** (Artane) or **benztropine mesylate** (Cogentin).

Tardive dyskinesia is characterized by abnormal involuntary movements frequently involving the facial, buccal, and masticatory muscles and often extending to the upper and lower extremities, including the neck, trunk, fingers, and toes. With continuous blockade, the dopaminergic receptors in the striatum upregulate. Following the discontinued use of neuroleptics or a reduction in dosage, the dyskinesia becomes

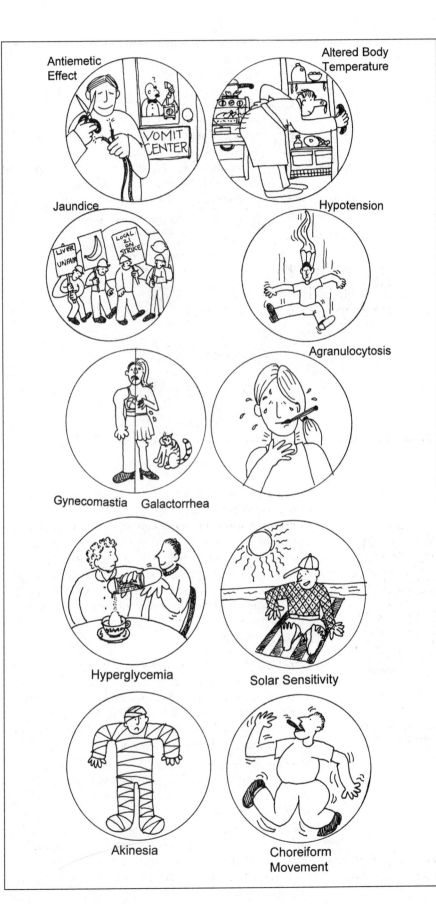

■**Fig. 7-5** ■
Effects and side effects of chlorpromazine.

apparent. The best prevention of tardive dyskinesia is to prescribe the neuroleptics at their lowest possible doses, have patients observe drug-free holidays, and avoid prescribing anticholinergic agents solely to prevent parkinsonism. See ■ **Fig. 7-5** ■

Neuroleptic Malignant Syndrome

Among the complications of neuroleptic chemotherapy, the most serious and potentially fatal complication is **malignant syndrome,** which is characterized by extreme hyperthermia; "lead pipe" skeletal muscle rigidity that causes dyspnea, dysphagia, and rhabdomyolysis; autonomic instability; fluctuating consciousness; leukocytosis; and elevated creatine phosphokinase levels.

The treatment of neuroleptic malignant syndrome consists of immediate discontinuation of the neuroleptic agent and administration of **dantrolene sodium** and dopamine function–enhancing substances such as **levodopa-carbidopa, bromocriptine,** or **amantadine.**

CHAPTER 8

Anxiolytic Agents

The anxiolytic agents consist of **benzodiazepine** derivatives and **azaspirodecanedione** derivatives.

This class of antianxiety agents shares the property of binding to a benzodiazepine receptor, part of the gamma aminobutyric acid (GABA) receptor-chloride channel complex whose function it modulates allosterically. Not only the anxiolytic effects of the benzodiazepines but also the **anticonvulsant, sedative,** or **muscle relaxant** effects seem to be mediated by the GABA-related mechanism. ■ **Fig. 8-1** ■

Besides the direct involvement of the GABA system, in parallel or more downstream to this, several other neurotransmitters such as **serotonin** have been suggested to participate in different aspects of benzodiazepine action. These anxioselectives include **buspirone, gepirone,** and **ipsapirone.**

Pharmacologic Properties of Benzodiazepine Derivatives

The pharmacology of benzodiazepine derivatives differs significantly from that of the neuroleptics, in that the benzodiazepines have no antipsychotic activity and cause no extrapyramidal, autonomic, or endocrine side effects. In addition, unlike the neuroleptics, which lower the seizure threshold, these substances are anticonvulsants. In addition, they are anxiolytics, muscle relaxants, and mild sedatives. Although the benzodiazepine derivatives do not produce pronounced autonomic or cardiovascular side effects, they can reduce or block the emotionally induced changes in cardiovascular functions, probably through actions on the limbic systems.

Compounds such as **oxazepam** and **lorazepam,** which possess inactive metabolites, are relatively short acting, whereas compounds such as **prazepam,** with several active metabolites, have longer disposition half-lives. Consequently, it may be necessary to reduce the doses of those benzodiazepines with active metabolites.

Mode of Action of Benzodiazepine Derivatives

Antianxiety Effects

Benzodiazepines, by facilitating GABAergic actions, exert their anxiety-reducing effects by depressing the hyperactivity of neuronal circuits in the limbic system. In addition, they may inhibit the hyperexcitability of hippocampal cholinergic and serotonergic neurons. See ■ **Fig. 8-1** ■

Muscle Relaxant Activity

Benzodiazepines enhance presynaptic inhibition by releasing GABA from interneurons and by facilitating the action of glycine in the spinal cord and brainstem. Glutamate and aspartate have excitatory effects on neurons, whereas **GABA, glycine,** and **taurine** have inhibitory actions in the CNS.

Sedative Effects

The sleep-promoting effects of benzodiazepines may relate to their ability to reduce hyperarousability and emotional tension. The **anterograde amnesia** produced by high doses may be due to their interference with hippocampal functions. See ■ **Fig. 8-1** ■

Anticonvulsant Activity

Benzodiazepine derivatives are thought to exert their anticonvulsant activity by facilitating GABAergic transmission. Substances that inhibit the synthesis of GABA (e.g., **isoniazid**) or block the GABA recognition site (e.g., **bicuculline**) cause convulsions. See ■ **Figs. 6-1 and 6-11** ■

Therapeutic Uses of Benzodiazepines

Neurotic Anxiety States

Benzodiazepines are of value in the treatment of **anxious depression** and anxiety-tension associated with schizophrenia, as well as in patients undergoing psychotherapy. They should be used only

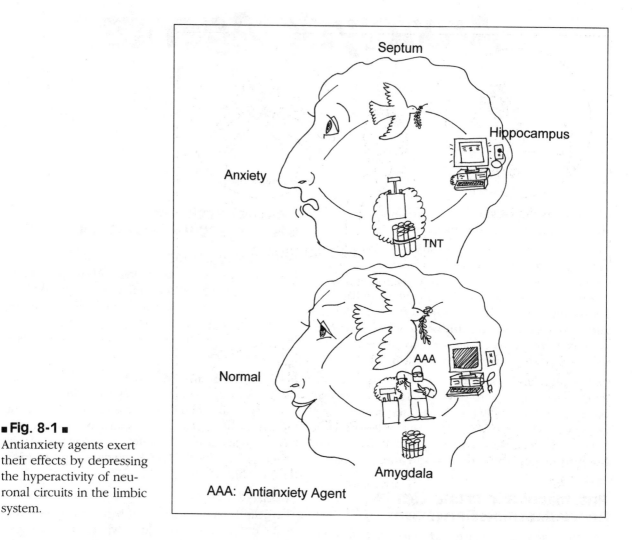

■ Fig. 8-1 ■
Antianxiety agents exert their effects by depressing the hyperactivity of neuronal circuits in the limbic system.

(Figure labels: Septum, Hippocampus, Anxiety, TNT, Normal, AAA, Amygdala, AAA: Antianxiety Agent)

when the symptoms are disabling, not just to alleviate stress. **■ Fig. 8-2 ■**

Neuromuscular Disorders

Benzodiazepines are of value in alleviating the symptoms of **cerebral palsy,** spasticity resulting from degenerative disorders such as **multiple sclerosis, tetanus, stiff-man syndrome,** and backache and muscle strain. The effective dosages are generally large and may be increased as the disease progresses (e.g., multiple sclerosis). See **■ Fig. 8-2 ■**

Intractable Seizures

To abort an epileptic seizure, **diazepam,** given intravenously, is a drug of choice. **Clonazepam** is also effective See **■ Fig. 8-2 ■**

Alcohol Withdrawal

During acute withdrawal from alcohol, the IV administration of **diazepam** is recommended, usually followed by **chlordiazepoxide** given orally. See **■ Fig. 8-2 ■**

Sleep Disorders

Diazepam and **flunitrazepam** are often used as sedatives. In addition, these agents are effective in controlling somnambulism, enuresis, and night terrors.

Preanesthetic Medications and Diagnostic Procedures

Intravenously administered **diazepam** may be used for induction prior to maintaining anesthesia with other agents, in endoscopic procedures, and in cardioversion. In general these agents cause amnesia, relieve anxiety, and reduce or eliminate the use of narcotic analgesics. During labor and delivery, only short-acting benzodiazepines such as **oxazepam** should be used. See **■ Fig. 8-2 ■**

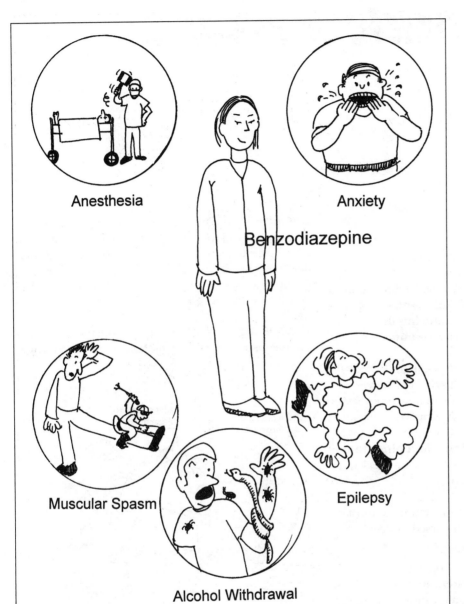

Anesthesia

Anxiety

Benzodiazepine

Muscular Spasm

Alcohol Withdrawal

Epilepsy

■Fig. 8-2 ■
Therapeutic usefulness of
benzodiazepine derivatives.

Unwanted Side Effects and Hazards

The most troublesome side effects associated with many of the anxiolytic agents are **drowsiness** and **postural hypotension,** which may be especially pronounced in elderly patients. In children, benzodiazepines should be limited to the management of convulsive disorders. Because benzodiazepines are metabolized extensively, they should be used with extreme caution in patients suffering from liver diseases.

CHAPTER 9

Antidepressants

Classification of Antidepressants

Antidepressants are divided into three classes:

1. **Dibenzapine derivatives,** called **tricyclic antidepressants.** They include **imipramine** (Tofranil), **desipramine** (Norpramin), **amitriptyline** (Elavil), **nortriptyline** (Aventyl), **protriptyline** (Vivactil), and **doxepin** (Adapin).
2. **Monoamine oxidase inhibitors,** used occasionally to treat depression. The **hydrazine** derivatives consist of **isocarboxazid** (Marplan) and **phenelzine sulfate** (Nardil). The **nonhydrazine** derivatives include **tranylcypromine** (Parnate).
3. Newer agents: **amoxapine, doxepin, fluoxetine, maprotiline, trazodone, mianserin, alprazolam,** and **bupropion.**

Because the tricyclic antidepressants are the most often used drugs, they will be discussed in detail.

Tricyclic Antidepressants

Tricyclic antidepressants, like some of the phenothiazine derivatives, are **sedative in nature.** Those compounds containing a **tertiary amine** (imipramine, amitriptyline, and doxepin) are the most sedative. Compounds containing a **secondary amine** (nortriptyline and desipramine) are less so, and protriptyline has no sedative effect.

Tricyclic antidepressants, like some of the phenothiazine derivatives (e.g., **thoriodazine**), have an **anticholinergic property. Amitriptyline** is the strongest and **desipramine** the weakest in this regard.

The tricyclic antidepressants also have **cardiovascular actions.** In particular, they cause orthostatic hypotension by obtunding the various reflex mechanisms involved in maintaining blood pressure.

Antidepressants may block the **uptake of norepinephrine or serotonin.** ■ **Fig. 9-1** ■

Side Effects - The first-generation tricyclic antidepressants, the monoamine oxidase inhibitors, and the newer agents can cause sedation, insomnia, orthostatic hypotension, or nausea. Because of their anticholinergic properties, they may also produce cardiac toxicities. ■ **Fig. 9-2** ■

Therapeutic Indications - A primary indication for the use of tricyclic antidepressants is **endoge-**

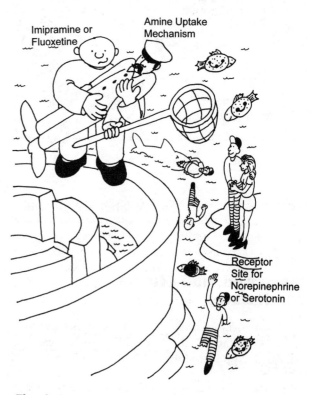

■Fig. 9-1 ■
Imipramine and fluoxetine exert their antidepressant actions in part by blocking the uptake of norepinephrine and serotonin.

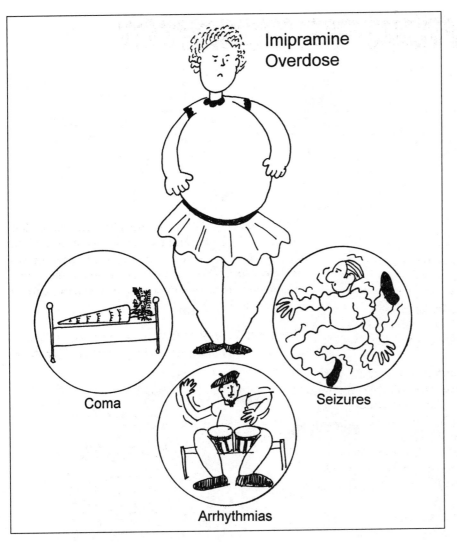

Imipramine
Overdose

Coma

Seizures

Arrhythmias

■ Fig. 9-2 ■
Toxic effects of
imipramine.

nous depression. ■ **Fig. 9-3** ■ The effective dosage of tricyclic antidepressants, which are equivalent drugs, is chosen empirically. The less sedative agents are chosen for apathetic and withdrawn patients. Because the **margin of safety** for these agents is narrow, they should not be prescribed in large quantities for a depressed patient who may use them to attempt suicide.

The anticholinergic effect of **imipramine** has been used successfully in managing **enuresis. ■ Fig. 9-4; see Fig. 9-3** ■

The **pain** associated with diabetic peripheral neuropathy, trigeminal neuralgia, or cancer may predispose such patients to depression. Tricyclic antidepressants have been shown to be an effective

adjunct in managing these and other similar conditions. See ■ **Fig. 9-3** ■

Some episodic **phobias** are regarded as "masked" depression and thus respond to treatment with tricyclic antidepressants. See ■ **Fig. 9-3** ■

Fluoxetine, in addition to its antidepressant property, has been used as an **appetite suppressant. Imipramine** and **desipramine** have been used as **antibulimic substances.**

Desipramine has been used as part of the treatment of **alcoholism.** Because depression has led to relapsed drinking in alcoholics striving to maintain sobriety, treatment with antidepressants may reverse or prevent these depressive symptoms.

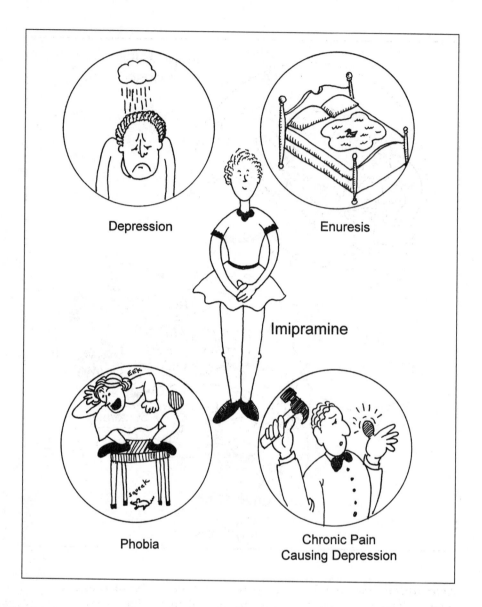

■Fig. 9-3 ■
Therapeutic uses of
imipramine.

Fatal Overdoses - The diagnostic triad of **coma, seizures,** and **cardiac arrhythmias** should raise the suspicion of tricyclic overdose. See **■ Fig. 9-2 ■** A trial dose of IV-administered **physostigmine** (1–4 mg) may suggest the diagnosis because this will awaken the comatose patient or mitigate the arrhythmias.

Monoamine Oxidase Inhibitors

In general, not only do these agents inhibit the oxidase that metabolizes amines **■ Figs. 9-5 and 9-6 ■** but they also inhibit the oxidase that metabolizes drugs and essential nutrients. Hence, the incidence of drug-drug and drug-food interactions is extremely high with these agents. **■ Fig. 9-7 ■**

These agents are used for patients who have not responded to a tricyclic antidepressant for an adequate trial period and with an appropriate dosage; who have developed allergic reactions to tricyclics; or who have had previous depressive episodes that responded well to monoamine oxidase inhibitors.

Newer Antidepressants

The newer agents that may have actions that are novel or atypical include maprotiline, amoxapine, fluoxetine, trazodone, bupropion, mianserin, and alprazolam.

Maprotiline has relatively minor anticholinergic properties compared to amitriptyline. It has a very large elimination half-life of 36–48 hours. In large doses it produces convulsions.

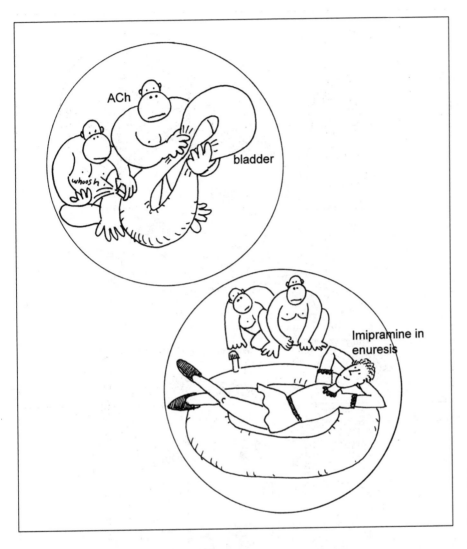

■Fig. 9-4 ■
The anticholinergic property of imipramine is beneficial in treating enuresis.

Amoxapine has neuroleptic properties that stem from its dopamine receptor-binding affinity. Similar to the neuroleptics, it may produce movement disorders. In toxic doses, amoxapine may provoke difficult-to-control convulsions.

Fluoxetine selectively blocks the uptake of serotonin. It is devoid of anticholinergic properties and hence has little or no effect on the cardiovascular system, including orthostatic hypotension or arrhythmias.

Trazodone is perhaps the most sedative antidepressant available. It is devoid of anticholinergic effects and causes postural hypotension as well as rarely serious **priapism.**

Bupropion is free of anticholinergic, antiadrenergic, and cardiotoxic properties. Its structure is related to that of amphetamine, and it possesses stimulating effects; hence it may be useful in hyperphagic or obese individuals.

Mianserin does not alter the uptake of norepinephrine, serotonin, or dopamine. It is devoid of anticholinergic properties and thus is not cardiotoxic. It blocks both alpha$_1$- and alpha$_2$-adrenergic receptors, and mianserin is sedative in nature.

Alprazolam causes pronounced sedation but is devoid of anticholinergic properties. Alprazolam and, to a certain extent, clonazepam are effective in the treatment of panic disorder.

Control of Manic Episodes in Manic-Depressive Psychosis Using Lithium

Because lithium is not bound to any plasma or tissue proteins, it is widely distributed throughout the body.
■ Fig. 9-8 ■

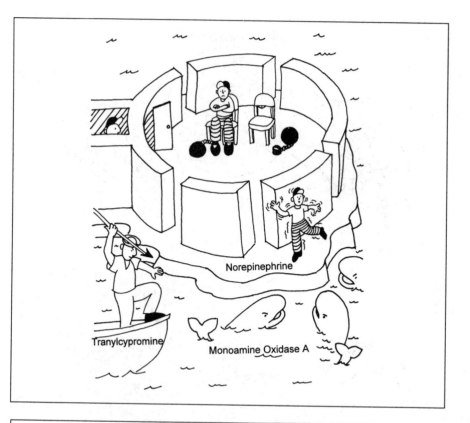

■Fig. 9-5 ■
Norepinephrine and serotonin are metabolized by monoamine oxidase A.

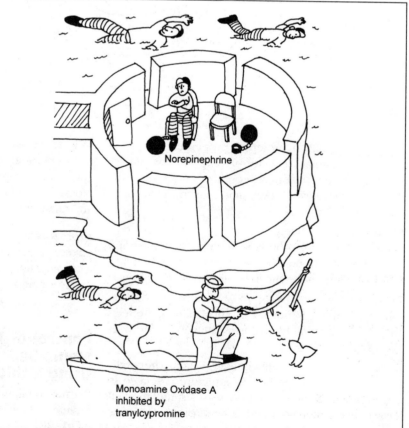

■Fig. 9-6 ■
Tranylcypromine inhibits the activity of monoamine oxidase A.

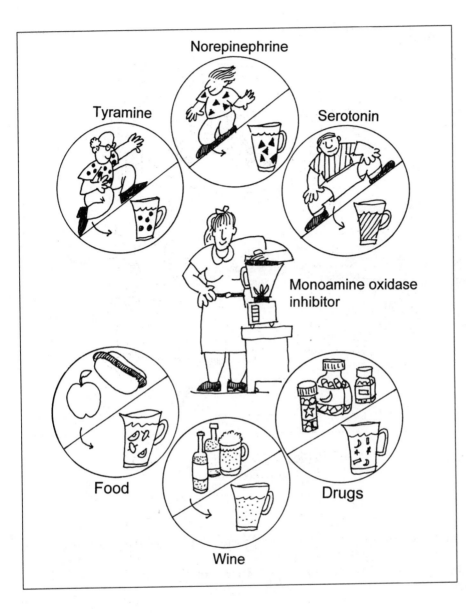

Norepinephrine

Tyramine

Serotonin

Monoamine oxidase
inhibitor

Food

Drugs

Wine

■ **Fig. 9-7** ■
In addition to metabolizing
amines, monoamine oxi-
dases are also involved in
metabolizing drugs and
food products.

Lithium ions are **eliminated** mainly by the kidneys. There is a direct relationship between the amount of **sodium chloride** ingested and the fraction of filtered lithium resorbed; the lower the sodium intake, the greater is the lithium retention. The **contraindications** are significant cardiovascular or renal diseases that would compromise its excretion. ■ **Fig. 9-9** ■

Side Effects

When the maintenance dosage of lithium is being established, the patient may experience **GI discom-** forts, such as nausea, vomiting, diarrhea, stomach pain, muscular weakness, unusual thirst, frequent urination, a slight feeling of being dazed, fatigue, and sleepiness. These early side effects disappear once the patient is stabilized.

From the beginning of treatment, patients exhibit slight and barely noticeable **hand tremors,** which do not respond to antiparkinsonian agents.

After several months of continuous therapy with lithium, patients may develop **diabetes insipidus** and **goiter.** The kidney tubules then become insensi-

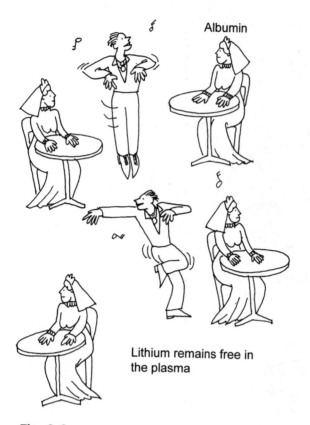

Albumin

Lithium remains free in
the plasma

Fig. 9-8
Lack of binding of lithium to plasma
proteins.

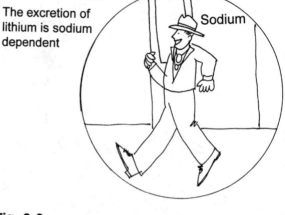

Lithium only

The excretion of
lithium is sodium
dependent

Sodium

Fig. 9-9
Sodium-dependent excretion of lithium.

tive to the action of **antidiuretic hormone,** and its administration is ineffective. Either a dose reduction or discontinuation of the lithium corrects this side effect without leaving any residual pathology. In the presence of goiter, the patient remains euthyroid. It has been reported that the administration of small amounts of **thyroxine** may counteract this side effect. ■ **Fig. 9-10** ■

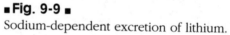

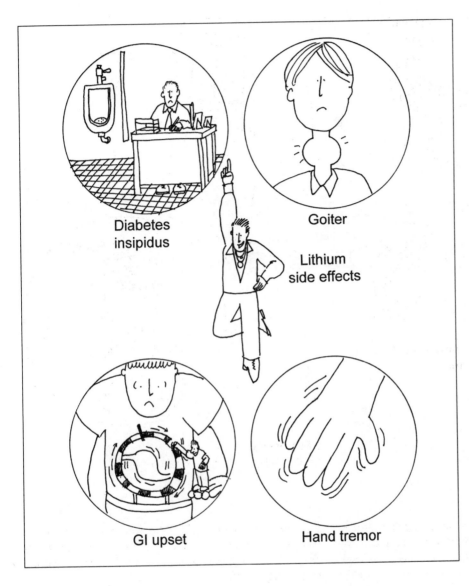

Diabetes insipidus

Goiter

Lithium side effects

GI upset

Hand tremor

■Fig. 9-10 ■
Side effects of lithium.

V

Central Nervous System Pharmacology

CHAPTER 10

Narcotic Analgesics

Analgesia means lack of pain, and **analgesics** are substances that obtund the perception of pain without causing loss of consciousness.

Morphine

Effects on the Central Nervous System

Morphine, a naturally occurring analgesic, depresses the cerebral cortex, hypothalamus, and medullary centers. These effects are responsible for suppressing pain perception, inducing narcosis, depressing the cough center, depressing the vomiting center, and depressing respiration.

Initially morphine stimulates the vomiting center, and emesis occurs early in cases of intoxication. Depression of the vomiting center then ensues late in intoxication. Morphine stimulates the vagus nerve, causing **bradycardia,** and stimulates the nucleus of the third cranial nerve (oculomotor), causing **miosis.** ■ **Fig. 10-1** ■

Analgesic Effects

Morphine exerts its analgesic effects by elevating the pain threshold and, especially, by altering the patient's reactions to pain.

Therapeutic Uses

In a relatively small dose of 5–10 mg, morphine relieves the constant but dull pain originating from the viscera, such as that of coronary, pulmonary, and biliary origin. In somewhat larger doses (10–20 mg), morphine relieves the sharp, lancinating, and intermittent pain resulting from bone fractures and other physical injuries. Inoperable and terminal causes of neoplastic diseases usually require the administration of morphine or other narcotics in increasing doses that eventually lead to both tolerance and addiction.

Effects of Morphine

Depression of Respiration - Morphine depresses all phases of respiration (respiratory rate, tidal volume, and minute volume) when given in subhyp-

notic and subanalgesic doses. In humans, a morphine overdose causes respiratory arrest and death.

Effects on the Cardiovascular System - Morphine releases **histamine** and may cause peripheral vasodilation and orthostatic hypotension. See ■ **Fig. 10-1** ■ The cutaneous blood vessels dilate around the "blush areas," such as the face, neck, and upper thorax. Morphine causes cerebral vasodilation (due to increased carbon dioxide retention secondary to respiratory depression), and hence it increases the cerebrospinal fluid pressure. Therefore, morphine should be used cautiously in patients with either meningitis or recent head injury. When given subcutaneously, morphine is absorbed poorly whenever there is either traumatic or hemorrhagic shock.

Effects on the Gastrointestinal Tract - Morphine reduces the activity of the entire GI tract in that it reduces the secretion of hydrochloric acid, diminishes the motility of the stomach, and increases the tone of the upper part of the duodenum. These actions may delay passage of the stomach contents into the duodenum. That both pancreatic and biliary secretions are diminished may also hinder digestion. In the large intestine, the propulsive peristaltic wave in the colon is reduced, the muscle tone including that of the anal sphincter is increased, and the gastrocolic reflex (defecation reflex) is reduced. These actions, in combination, cause constipation, which seems to be a chronic problem among addicts. ■ **Fig. 10-2** ■

Antidiarrheal Effects - Opiate preparations, usually given as **paregoric,** are effective and fast-acting antidiarrheal agents. These agents are also useful postoperatively to produce solid stool following an **ileostomy** or **colostomy**.

Oliguric Effect - Morphine causes oliguria and this results from (1) pronounced diaphoresis, (2) the relative hypotension and decreased glomerular filtration rate, and (3) the release of antidiuretic hormone from the neurohypophysis. In an elderly patient with prostatic hypertrophy, morphine may cause acute uri-

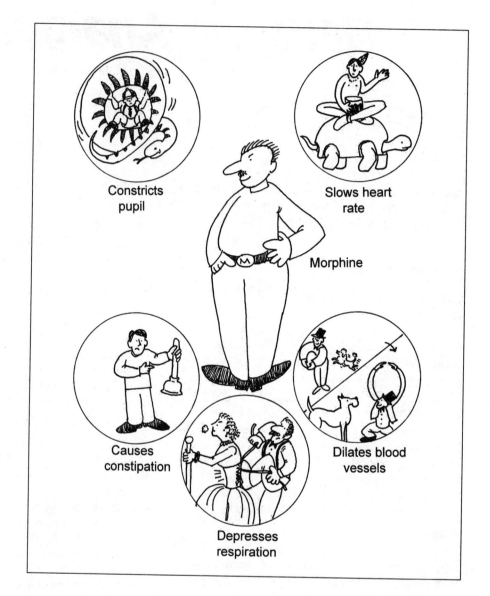

■ Fig. 10-1 ■
Pharmacologic actions of
morphine.

nary retention. Morphine may reduce the effectiveness of a diuretic when both drugs are used in combination in the treatment of congestive heart failure.

Codeine

Unlike morphine, codeine is **absorbed orally.** The
side effects are the same as morphine's but are milder
and far less frequent.

The Synthetic Analgesics

Meperidine

The pharmacology of meperidine resembles that of
morphine, with the following exceptions. The anti-

tussive and antidiarrheal effects of meperidine are
minimal. Meperidine does not produce miosis and
may even cause mydriasis. Meperidine's **duration of
action** is extremely short, and hence it is used as an
analgesic during diagnostic procedures such as cys-
toscopy, gastroscopy, pneumoencephalography, and
retrograde pyelography. It is also used as a **preanesthetic medication** and an **obstetric analgesic**. See
■ Fig. 10-2 ■

Methadone

Pharmacologically, methadone is very similar to morphine, with the following exceptions. Methadone is
effective orally. Its onset and duration of action are

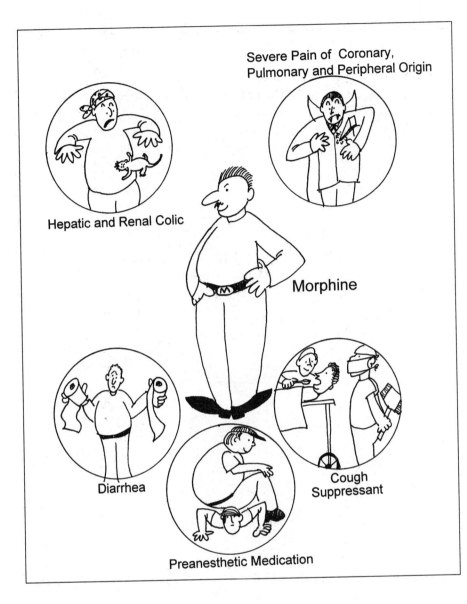

Severe Pain of Coronary,
Pulmonary and Peripheral Origin

Hepatic and Renal Colic

Morphine

Diarrhea

Cough
Suppressant

Preanesthetic Medication

■Fig. 10-2 ■
Therapeutic uses of morphine.

longer than morphine's. **Tolerance** to methadone develops very slowly, and if it is abruptly withdrawn, the abstinence syndrome develops more slowly, is less intense, and is more prolonged than the abstinence syndrome of morphine. The **abuse potential** of methadone is lower than morphine's.

Like morphine, methadone is used in the management of pain. It is also used in the detoxification and treatment of narcotic addiction.

Dextropropoxyphene

Dextropropoxyphene is an analgesic with a potency two-thirds that of codeine.

Opioids with Mixed Actions: Agonist-Antagonists and Partial Agonists

Pentazocine (Talwin)

The analgesia produced by 30 mg of pentazocine, **a mixed-narcotic agonist and a weak antagonist,** is comparable to that elicited by 10 mg of morphine. Its onset and duration of action are shorter than those of morphine. Pentazocine will antagonize some of the respiratory depression and analgesia produced by morphine and meperidine. However, the analgesic action and respiratory depression produced by pentazocine can be reversed by a narcotic antagonist.

Pentazocine causes tolerance and addiction, but their emergences are very slow compared to those induced by morphine.

Opioid Receptor Antagonists

Naloxone (Narcan) and **naltrexone hydrochloride** (Trexan) reverse the respiratory-depressant action of the narcotics related to morphine, meperidine, and methadone. Naloxone neither antagonizes the respiratory-depressant effects of barbiturates and other hypnotics nor aggravates their depressant effects on respiration.

Antitussive Preparations

Dextromethorphan (Romilar) exerts no depressant effects on respiration and lacks addiction liability. It is an antitussive agent with a potency approximately one-half that of codeine.

CHAPTER 11

Analgesics-Antipyretics and Antiinflammatory Agents

Salicylates and allied compounds have **analgesic, antipyretic, uricosuric,** and **antiinflammatory** properties. Their mechanisms of action differ from those of the antiinflammatory steroids and the opioid analgesics.

The pharmacology of acetysalicylic acid (aspirin) is discussed in detail as a prototype drug, and all the other drugs are compared to it.

The mechanism by which these drugs act to reduce mild to moderate pain is based on the relationship between drugs such as aspirin and **prostaglandin** synthesis. Studies in humans have shown that IV administration of certain prostaglandins elicits headache and pain and produces hyperalgesia, sensitizing the individual to stimuli that normally would not produce pain. Aspirin and related compounds inhibit the enzyme **cyclooxygenase** and prevent the formation of **prostaglandin.**

Aspirin and Its Uses

Aspirin-Induced Analgesia

Aspirin does not depress respiration, is relatively nontoxic, and lacks addiction liability. Aspirin is a weak or mild analgesic that is effective for ameliorating short, intermittent types of pain such as neuralgia, myalgia, and toothache. ■ **Fig. 11-1** ■ It does not have the efficacy of morphine and cannot relieve the severe, prolonged, and lancinating types of pain associated with such trauma as burns or fractures. Like morphine, it produces analgesia by raising the pain threshold in the thalamus, but, unlike morphine, it does not alter the patient's reactions to pain. Because aspirin does not cause hypnosis or euphoria, its site of action has been postulated to be subcortical. In addition to **raising the pain threshold,** the antiinflammatory effects of aspirin may contribute to its analgesic actions.

Aspirin-Induced Antipyresis

Aspirin acts by causing cutaneous **vasodilation,** which prompts perspiration and enhances heat dissipation. See ■ **Fig. 11-1** ■

Uricosuric Effects

Small doses (600 mg) of aspirin cause **hyperuricemia,** but large doses (>5 g) have a uricosuric effect. Aspirin inhibits uric acid resorption by the tubules in the kidneys.

Antiinflammatory Effects

Aspirin has an **antiinflammatory** action as well as **antirheumatic** and **antiarthritic** effects and therefore may be used in the treatment of rheumatic fever. Aspirin is extremely effective in managing rheumatoid arthritis and allied diseases involving the joints, such as anklyosing spondylitis and osteoarthritis. It is thought that aspirin and indomethacin exert their antiinflammatory effects by inhibiting **prostaglandin** synthesis through the inhibition of **cyclooxygenase.** The presynthesized prostaglandins are released during a tissue injury that fosters inflammation and pain. Furthermore, aspirin reduces the formation of prostaglandin in the platelets and leukocytes, which is responsible for the reported hematologic effects associated with aspirin. See ■ **Fig. 11-1** ■

Cardiovascular Disease

The current thinking concerning the role of aspirin in the prevention of cardiovascular disease is that it is beneficial in the event of **myocardial infarction** and **stroke.** It is effective because, in platelets, small amounts of aspirin acetylate irreversibly and bind to the active site of **thromboxane A_2,** a potent promoter of **platelet aggregation.** See ■ **Fig. 11-1** ■

Premenstrual Syndrome

The menstrual cycle is associated with two potentially incapacitating events: **dysmenorrhea** and the **premenstrual syndrome.** Substantial evidence indicates that the excessive production of prostaglandin F_{2a} is the major source of painful menstruation. The nonsteroidal antiinflammatory drugs approved for the treatment of dysmenorrhea are **aspirin, ibuprofen, mefenamic acid,** and **naproxen.**

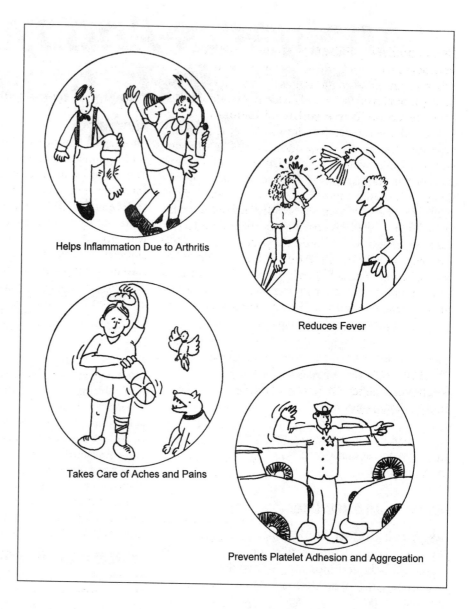

Helps Inflammation Due to Arthritis

Reduces Fever

Takes Care of Aches and Pains

Prevents Platelet Adhesion and Aggregation

■**Fig. 11-1** ■
Therapeutic uses of aspirin.

Side Effects of Aspirin

Effects on Respiration - Aspirin both directly and indirectly stimulates respiration. In toxic doses, it causes hyperventilation and respiratory alkalosis. If the salicylate level continues to rise, it may cause respiratory acidosis and metabolic acidosis.

Aspirin Poisoning - The supportive treatment of aspirin poisoning may include **gastric lavage** (to prevent the further absorption of salicylate), **fluid replenishment** (to offset the dehydration and oliguria), **alcohol and water sponging** (to combat the hyperthermia), the administration of **vitamin K** (to prevent possible hemorrhage), **sodium bicarbo-** **nate** administration (to combat acidosis), and, in extreme cases, **peritoneal dialysis** and **exchange transfusion.**

Gastrointestinal Effects - Although innocuous in most subjects, the therapeutic analgesic doses of aspirin may cause epigastric distress, nausea, vomiting, and bleeding. Aspirin can also exacerbate the symptoms of peptic ulcer, characterized by heartburn, dyspepsia, and erosive gastritis. Furthermore, compounds possessing antiinflammatory properties (**aspirin, phenylbutazone,** and **oxyphenbutazone**) are associated with a higher incidence of GI toxicity than those compounds devoid of antiinflammatory properties (**phenacetin** and **acetaminophen**).

Hematopoietic Effects - Aspirin reduces the **leukocytosis** associated with acute rheumatic fever. When given on a long-term basis, it also reduces the hemoglobin level and the hematocrit. Aspirin use can cause reversible **hypoprothrombinemia** by interfering with the function of **vitamin K** in prothrombin synthesis. Therefore, aspirin should be used with caution in patients with vitamin K deficiency, preexisting hypoprothrombinemia, or hepatic damage; in patients taking anticoagulants; and in patients scheduled for surgery. Aspirin leads to **hemolytic anemia** in individuals with glucose-6-phosphate dehydrogenase deficiency. Aspirin prevents platelet aggregation and may be helpful in the treatment of thromboembolic diseases. See ■ **Fig. 11-1** ■ In addition to aspirin, indomethacin, phenylbutazone, sulfinpyrazone, and dipyridamole prevent platelet aggregation; in contrast, epinephrine, serotonin, and prostaglandins promote platelet aggregation and hence are procoagulants.

Treatment of Rheumatoid Arthritis and Degenerative Joint Disease

In the management of arthritic conditions, drugs are chosen on an empirical basis, with the least toxic substances being tried first. The following schedule may be used in drug selection, in the order listed:

1. Nonsteroidal antiinflammatory agents: Aspirin; ibuprofen, tolmetin, naproxen, fenoprofen, or sulindac; indomethacin or phenylbutazone
2. Disease-modifying agents: Gold salts, *d*-penicillamine, hydroxychloroquine
3. Steroids, immunosuppressive agents

Gold salt therapy is reserved for patients with progressive disease who do not obtain satisfactory relief from therapy with aspirin-like drugs. The principle that underlies this therapy is that gold, which accumulates in lysosomes, decreases the migration and phagocytic activity of macrophages. **Auroothioglucose, gold sodium thiomalate,** or **auranofin** may cause toxic effects such as cutaneous reactions (from erythema to exfoliative dermatitis) as well as albuminuria, hematuria, and thrombocytopenia.

Besides the nonsteroidal antiinflammatory agents and gold, other drugs are also used for the treatment of rheumatoid arthritis. These include immunosuppressive agents, glucocorticoids, penicillamine, and hydroxychloroquine. With the exception of glucocorticoids, these drugs resemble gold salts in that they do not possess antiinflammatory or analgesic properties, and

their therapeutic effects become evident only after several weeks or months of treatment.

Gout and Hyperuricemia

Allopurinol

Allopurinol (**Zyloprim**) reduces the synthesis of uric acid by inhibiting the activity of **xanthine oxidase.** The reduction in the uric acid pool occurs slowly. Because xanthine and hypoxanthine are more soluble than uric acid, they are easily excreted. Allopurinol is used not only in treating hyperuricemia associated with gout, but also in the secondary hyperuricemia associated with the use of antineoplastic agents. However, allopurinol may interfere with the metabolism of antineoplastic agents such as **azathioprine** and **6-mercaptopurine.**

Uricosuric Agents

The most commonly used uricosuric agents are **probenecid** (Benemid) and **sulfinpyrazone** (Anturane). In low doses, these agents block tubular secretion; at higher doses, they also block the tubular resorption of uric acid. Because the solubility of uric acid is increased in alkaline urine, the administration of sodium bicarbonate may at times be advantageous for offsetting this condition. In addition, probenecid and sulfinpyrazone inhibit the excretion of agents such as aspirin, penicillin, ampicillin, and indomethacin. Although probenecid and sulfinpyrazone may be coadministered, neither should be given with aspirin, which would nullify their uricosuric effects.

Treatment of an Acute Attack of Gout

Colchicine may be used diagnostically to ascertain the presence of gout and prophylactically to prevent its further occurrence. In addition to colchicine, phenylbutazone, indomethacin, corticotropin, and steroidal antiinflammatory agents may be used to treat the attack of gout.

Colchicine is tolerated well in moderate doses. Nausea, vomiting, diarrhea, and abdominal pain are the most common and earliest untoward effects of overdosage.

In the event of acute poisoning with colchicine, there is hemorrhagic gastroenteritis, extensive vascular damage, nephrotoxicity, muscular depression, and an ascending paralysis of the CNS.

Colchicine produces leukopenia that is soon replaced by leukocytosis.

The long-term administration of colchicine may lead to myopathy, neuropathy, agranulocytosis, aplastic anemia, alopecia, and azoospermia.

CHAPTER 12

General, Spinal, and Local Anesthetics

General Anesthetics

Anesthesia is the controllable and reversible depression of the CNS and is characterized by a lack of perception of all sensations, by **analgesia,** and by **amnesia.**

Because general anesthetics alter the **cardiac and respiratory physiology,** those agents causing myocardial irritability, hypotension, circulatory depression, or tachyarrhythmia should be used with extreme caution in patients who have preexisting cardiovascular problems. Furthermore, agents causing **respiratory depression** should be used with caution in patients with bronchitis, emphysema, muscular dystrophy, or myasthenia gravis, as well as in those in bronchospastic states. The use of **skeletal muscle relaxants** should be monitored in conditions of respiratory insufficiency such as **kyphoscoliosis.** The opioids, which further depress respiration, should also be used with extreme care. ■ **Fig. 12-1** ■

Preanesthetic Medications

The preanesthetic medications are given for the following reasons:

- To sedate and reduce anxiety (secobarbital, diazepam)
- To relieve pain, if present (opioids)
- To reduce excess salivation (anticholinergics such as atropine)
- To prevent bradycardia during surgery (atropine)
- To facilitate intubation (succinylcholine) ■ **Fig. 12-2** ■

Classification of General Anesthetics

The general anesthetics are classified as inhalational or intravenous.

The **inhalational anesthetic agents** include:

Halogenated hydrocarbons
    Halothane

Anesthetic ethers
    Enflurane
    Isoflurane
    Methoxyflurane
Anesthetic gases
    Nitrous oxide

The **intravenous anesthetic agents** include:

Barbiturates
    Thiopental
    Methohexital
Nonbarbiturates
    Dissociative anesthetics (ketamine)
    Benzodiazepines (diazepam, midazolam, lorazepam)
    Neuroleptic anesthetics (droperidol, haloperidol)
    Imidazole derivatives (etomidate)
    Phenol derivatives (propofol)

Flumazenil blocks the actions of benzodiazepines.

Mode of Actions of the General Anesthetics

General anesthetics alter the **excitation of the neuronal membrane** and **modify impulse conduction.** They decrease the activity of neurons by increasing their threshold to fire. By interfering with sodium influx, they prevent the action potential from rising to a normal rate.

Signs and Stages of General Anesthesia

The **depth of anesthesia** is judged by the presence or absence of the eyelash reflex, the respiratory rate, and the response of the heart rate and blood pressure to surgical stimulation.

The various stages of anesthesia are: **Stage I** (analgesia), **Stage II** (excitement or delirium), **Stage III** (muscle relaxation and time of surgery), and **Stage IV** (death).

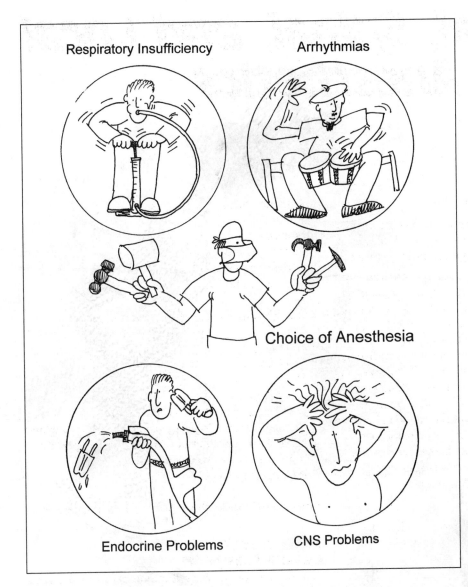

Fig. 12-1
Choice of anesthetics.

Factors Influencing Pharmacokinetics or Pharmacodynamics of General Anesthetics

The **administration of general anesthetics** is arbitrarily divided into three phases:

1. **Induction:** The time from the onset of administration of an anesthetic to a stage when surgery becomes suitable
2. **Maintenance:** The duration of time a patient is kept in a state of surgical anesthesia
3. **Emergence:** The time between the discontinuation of an anesthetic agent until the patient regains consciousness

The concentrations of general anesthetics in the brain depend on their **solubility,** their **concentration** in the inspired air, the **rate of pulmonary ventilation,** the **rate of pulmonary blood flow,** and the **concentration gradient** of the anesthetic between arterial and mixed venous blood. Furthermore, the greater the lipid solubility of an anesthetic, the lower the anesthetic tension needed to produce anesthesia. At equilibrium, the concentrations of an anesthetic in the brain and fat cells are high, but are low in the blood. Finally, the **potency** of an anesthetic is inversely related to its **minimum anesthetic concentration.**

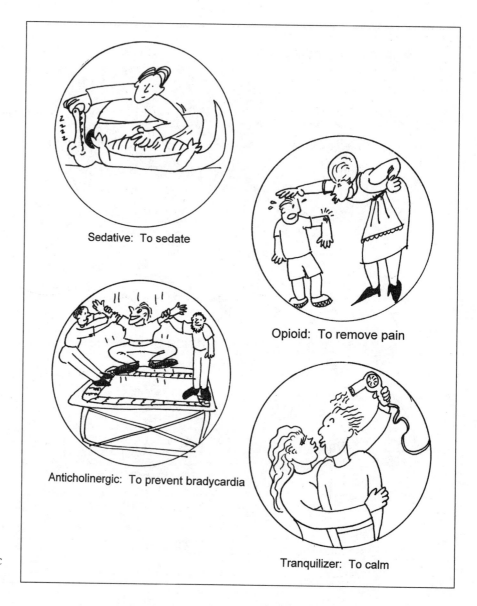

Sedative: To sedate

Opioid: To remove pain

Anticholinergic: To prevent bradycardia

Tranquilizer: To calm

■ Fig. 12-2 ■
Usefulness of preanesthetic
medications.

Spinal Anesthesia

Anesthesia of the lower extremities and abdomen
may be induced by the introduction of anesthetic
drugs into the subarachnoid space. The drug most often used for this purpose is **bupivacaine.**

The advantages of spinal anesthesia are the ease of
administration, rapid onset of anesthesia, and good
muscular relaxation. Additionally, it allows patients to
remain awake. **■ Fig. 12-3 ■**

The disadvantages of spinal anesthesia are hypotension (ephedrine and methoxamine may prevent this),
nausea and vomiting (avoided by thiopental), respiratory depression (treated by artificial respiration),
and postoperative headache (treated by increasing
the cerebrospinal fluid pressure). See **■ Fig. 12-3 ■**

Local Infiltration Anesthesia

General Pharmacology of Local Anesthetics

When a local anesthetic is injected near a nerve, it
blocks the flow of electrons along the axons and
eliminates the pain without loss of consciousness.
These effects are reversible. When administering a local anesthetic, one must remember that the larger the
diameter of the nerve fiber, the more anesthetic is
needed to produce anesthesia.

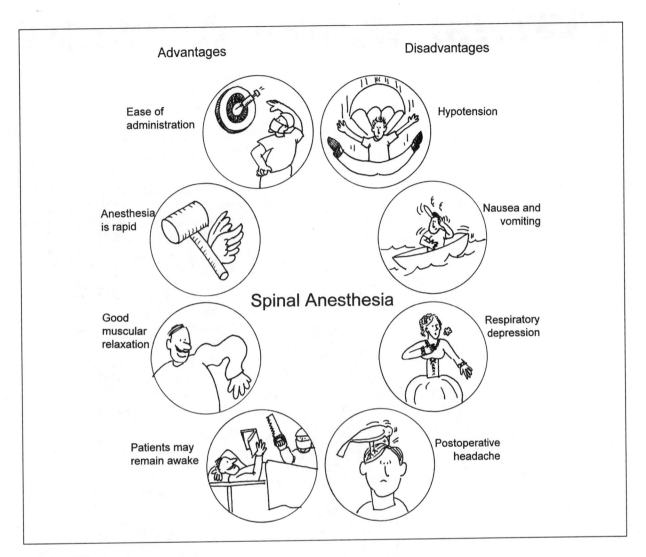

Advantages

Disadvantages

Ease of administration

Hypotension

Anesthesia is rapid

Nausea and vomiting

Spinal Anesthesia

Good muscular relaxation

Respiratory depression

Patients may remain awake

Postoperative headache

■Fig. 12-3 ■
Nature of spinal anesthesia.

Cocaine, procaine, chloroprocaine, and tetracaine are **"ester"**-containing anesthetics; whereas lidocaine, mepivacaine, prilocaine, bupivacaine, and etiocaine are **"amide"**-containing anesthetics.

Vascular Supply at the Site of Injection

Epinephrine is used in combination with a local anesthetic to reduce its uptake, prolong its duration of action, produce a bloodless field of operation, and protect against systemic effects.

Systemic Reactions

Cardiovascular Effects - Local anesthetics block the sodium channels, are cardiac depressants, and bring about a ventricular conduction defect and block that may progress to cardiac and ventilatory arrest if toxic doses are given. In addition, these agents produce arteriolar dilation.

Central Nervous System Effects - An overdose of local anesthetics can produce dose-dependent CNS side effects such as insomnia, visual and auditory disturbances, nystagmus, shivering, tonic-clonic convulsions, and fatal CNS depression.

Allergic Reactions - The **ester-containing local anesthetics** become metabolized to p-amino-benzoic acid derivatives, which have a potential for causing hypersensitivity reactions.

CHAPTER 13

Skeletal Muscle Relaxants

Neuromuscular blocking agents may be used to diagnose myasthenia gravis, facilitate endotracheal intubation, relieve laryngeal spasm, provide relaxation during brief diagnostic and surgical procedures, prevent bone fracture in electroconvulsive therapy, produce apnea and controlled ventilation during thoracic surgery and neurosurgery, reduce muscular spasticity in neurologic diseases (multiple sclerosis, cerebral palsy, or tetanus), and reduce the muscular spasm and pain resulting from sprains, arthritis, myositis, and fibrositis. ■ **Fig. 13-1** ■

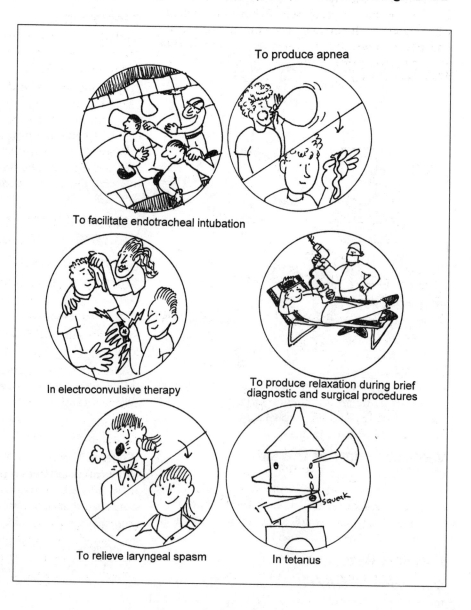

To produce apnea

To facilitate endotracheal intubation

In electroconvulsive therapy

To produce relaxation during brief diagnostic and surgical procedures

To relieve laryngeal spasm

In tetanus

■**Fig. 13-1** ■
Usefulness of neuromuscular blocking agents.

Skeletal muscle relaxants can be classified into four categories:

1. Depolarizing agents: Succinylcholine chloride (Anectine, Quelicin, Sux-Cert, Sucostrin)
2. Nondepolarizing or competitive-blocking agents: Tubocurarine chloride (Tubarine)
3. Direct-acting muscle relaxants: Dantrolene sodium (Dantrium)
4. Centrally acting muscle relaxants: Diazepam (Valium), baclofen (Lioresal)

Nicotinic Cholinergic Receptors

Acetylcholine and agents acting at the autonomic ganglia or the neuromuscular junctions interact with nicotinic cholinergic receptors to initiate the **end-plate potential** in muscle or an **excitatory postsynaptical potential** in nerve. ■ **Figs. 13-2 and 13-3** ■

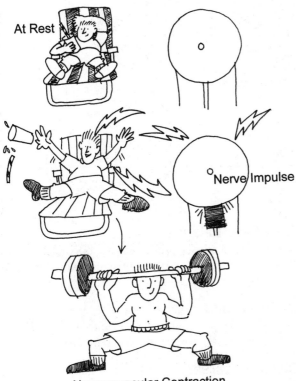

Neuromuscular Contraction

■**Fig. 13-2** ■
Acetylcholine causes muscular contraction.

Mechanism of Action of Neuromuscular Blocking Agents

Neuromuscular agents are classified as either **depolarizing agents** (e.g., succinylcholine) or **nondepolarizing agents** (e.g., tubocurarine). Succinylcholine has dual modes of action in that it possesses two phases of blocking action: depolarization and desensitization.

Agents such as **tubocurarine** and **pancuronium** compete with acetylcholine for the cholinergic receptors at the end plate. They combine with the receptors but do not activate them. Competitive or nondepolarizing agents are antagonized by neostigmine. ■ **Figs. 13-4 and 13-5** ■

Dantrolene

Dantrolene is thought to reduce the amount of **calcium** released and, hence, to prevent excitation-contraction coupling.

The sequence of and onset of neuromuscular blockade is rapidly contracting muscles (eye, fingers, and toes) followed by slowly contracting muscles (diaphragm, limbs, and trunk). The onset and duration of action of succinylcholine are 1 and 5 minutes, respectively. The onset and duration of action of tubocurarine are 5 and 20 minutes, respectively.

Factors Affecting Neuromuscular Blockade

Drug Interactions

Antibiotics such as **neomycin** and **kanamycin** have been implicated as augmenting the action of the nondepolarizing agents.

Substances that **inhibit plasma cholinesterase** prolong the response of succinylcholine.

Antiarrhythmic agents such as **quinidine, procainamide,** and **propranolol** have been shown to augment *d*-tubocurarine-induced blockade.

Diuretics such as **thiazides, ethacrynic acid,** and **furosemide** intensify the effects of nondepolarizing muscle relaxants.

The **local anesthetics procaine** and **lidocaine** enhance the neuromuscular block produced by nondepolarizing and depolarizing muscle relaxants.

Calcium ions play an important role in the presynaptic release of acetylcholine, and prolonged neuromuscular blockade has been reported after calcium antagonist administration during anesthesia that

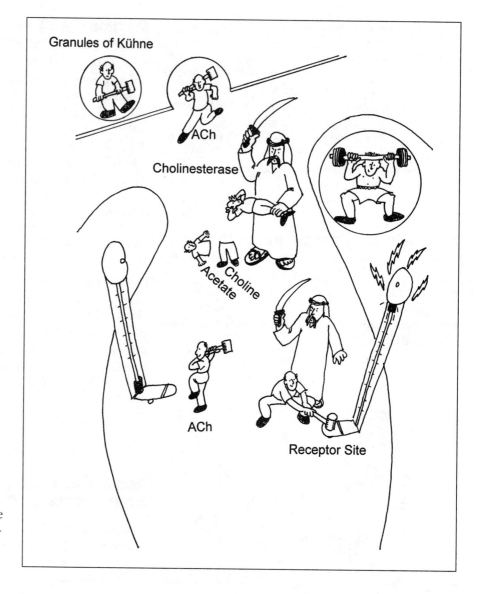

Granules of Kühne

ACh

Cholinesterase

Acetate

Choline

ACh

Receptor Site

■ **Fig. 13-3** ■

The action of acetylcholine at the neuromuscular junction is terminated by acetylcholinesterase.

includes concurrent nondepolarizing neuromuscular blockade. **Ketamine** potentiates neuromuscular blockade produced by tubocurarine but not that produced by succinylcholine.

Electrolytes

Diuretic-induced chronic hypokalemia reduces the pancuronium requirements for neuromuscular blockade, and thus more neostigmine is required to achieve antagonism.

The dose of a muscle relaxant should be reduced in patients who have **toxemia** associated with **pregnancy** and are undergoing **magnesium** replacement therapy.

Acid-Base Balance

Respiratory acidosis enhances d-tubocurarine- and pancuronium-induced neuromuscular block and opposes reversal by neostigmine.

Hypothermia

Hypothermia prolongs the neuromuscular blockade produced by d-tubocurarine and pancuronium.

Disease States

The plasma concentrations of d-tubocurarine and pancuronium are increased in patients with impaired liver functions because liver disease interferes with the metabolism of pancuronium.

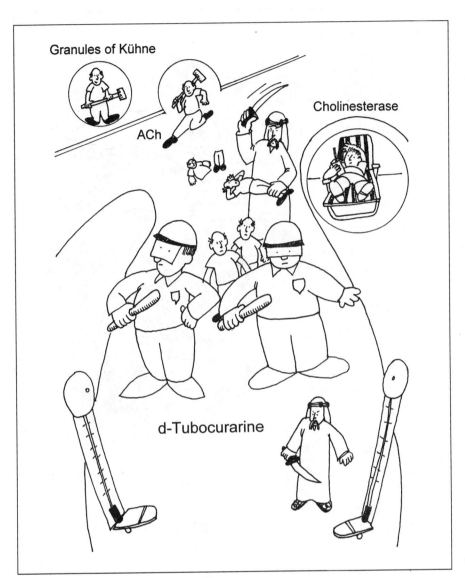

Granules of Kühne

ACh

Cholinesterase

d-Tubocurarine

■**Fig. 13-4** ■
d-Tubocurarine competes with the action of acetyl-choline.

Age

Neonates are more sensitive to nondepolarizing muscle relaxants. The response of small infants to some extent resembles that of adult patients with **myasthenia gravis**.

Side Effects of Neuromuscular Blocking Agents

Cardiovascular Effects

Succinylcholine may cause tachycardia, cardiac arrhythmias, and hypertension brought about by stimulation of the sympathetic ganglia. It may also provoke bradycardia, caused by stimulation of muscarinic receptor sites in the sinus node of the heart. This effect is more pronounced following a second dose of succinylcholine. The bradycardia may be blocked by thiopental, atropine, and ganglionic blocking agents.

Histamine Release

Tubocurarine and **succinylcholine** elicit histamine release in humans.

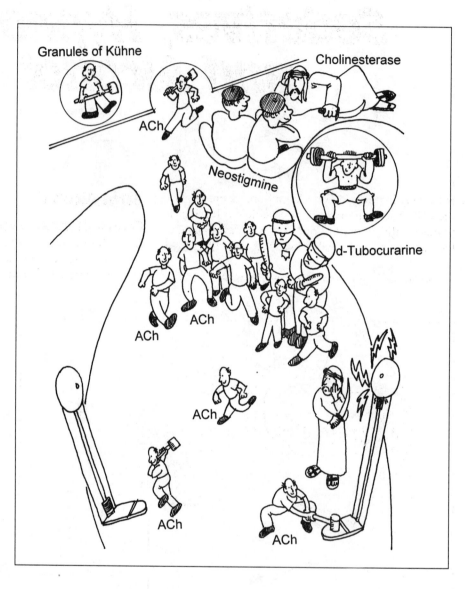

■Fig. 13-5 ■
Cholinesterase inhibitors,
which increase the level of
acetylcholine, reverse the
action of *d*-tubocurarine.

CHAPTER 14

Sedatives, Hypnotics, and Alcohol

Sedatives, hypnotics, and alcohol are depressants of the CNS. The degree of this reversible depression depends on the amount of drug ingested, producing effects according to the following scheme ■ **Fig. 14-1** ■:

Sedation → Hypnosis → Anesthesia → Death

Ethyl Alcohol

Central Nervous System Effects

As a CNS depressant, ethyl alcohol (**ethanol**) obeys the law of descending depression: it first inhibits the cerebral cortex, then the cerebellum, the spinal cord,

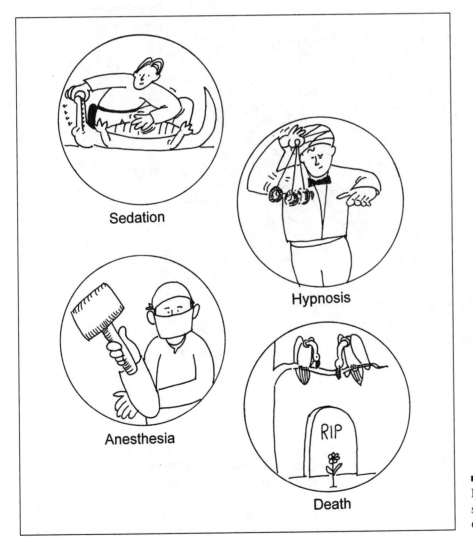

Sedation

Hypnosis

Anesthesia

Death

■**Fig. 14-1** ■
Dose-dependent depressant effect of drugs on the CNS.

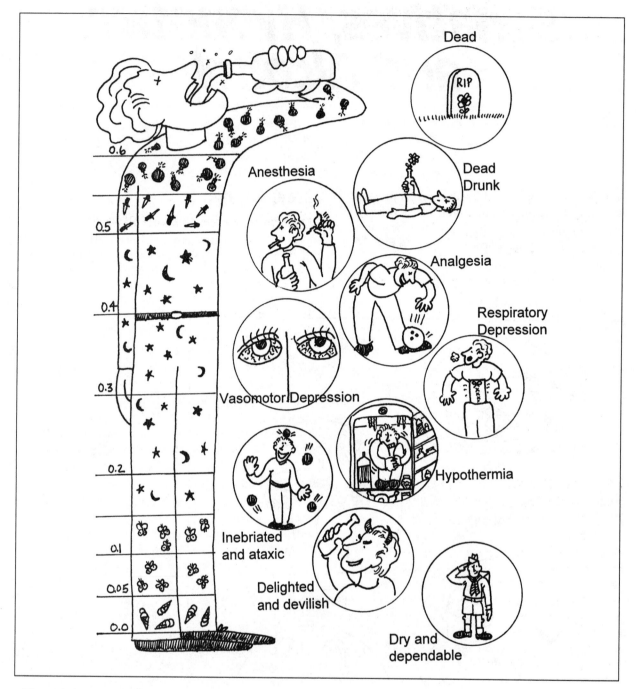

■Fig. 14-2 ■
Dose-dependent effects of ethanol.

and the medullary center. ■ **Fig. 14-2 ■ Death** is due to respiratory and cardiac failure.

Cardiovascular System Effects

Alcohol produces dilation of the skin vessels, flushing, and a sensation of warmth.

Gastrointestinal Effects

As a **gastric secretagogue,** alcohol stimulates the secretion of gastric juice, which is rich in acid and pepsin. Therefore, the consumption of alcohol is contraindicated in subjects with untreated **acid-pepsin disease.**

Liver Effects

Alcohol enhances the accumulation of fat in the liver.

Pharmacokinetics of Ethanol

The metabolism of ethanol, which shows genetic polymorphism, is catalyzed primarily by **alcohol dehydrogenase** with **zero-order kinetics,** according to the following scheme:

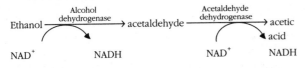

The rate-limiting factor in the metabolism of ethanol is the availability of NAD$^+$.

Methyl Alcohol Toxicology

Methyl alcohol is metabolized to **formaldehyde** and **formic acid,** according to the following reactions:

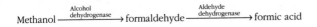

Methyl alcohol consumption leads to **acidosis** and **blindness.** The treatment of methyl alcohol poisoning may include water and electrolyte replacement along with the administration of sodium bicarbonate to combat the acidosis. Ethyl alcohol may also be administered intravenously because it is a preferred substrate by liver alcohol dehydrogenase, thus allowing methyl alcohol to be excreted unmetabolized in the urine.

Sedatives and Hypnotics

Sedatives and hypnotics may be divided into two categories: barbiturates and nonbarbiturates.

The Barbiturates

The primary mechanism of action of barbiturates is to increase inhibition of neurons through the **gamma-aminobutyric acid** system. Anesthetic barbiturates also decrease excitation via a decrease in calcium conductance.

Classification

Barbiturates are classified according to their **duration of action:**

- **Ultra-short-acting** (thiopental and methohexital)
- **Short- to intermediate-acting** (pentobarbital, secobarbital, and amobarbital)
- **Long-acting** (phenobarbital)

Barbiturates do not raise the **pain threshold** and have no **analgesic** property.

Pharmacokinetics

They are metabolized in the liver by aliphatic oxygenation, aromatic oxygenation, and *N*-dealkylation.

The inactive metabolites are excreted in the urine. The administration of **bicarbonate** enhances the urinary excretion of barbiturates that have a pK_a of 7.4 (phenobarbital and thiopental). This generalization is not true of other barbiturates. The long-term administration of barbiturates activates the cytochrome P-450 drug metabolizing system (see Chap. 1).

Acute Toxicity

The treatment of poisoning consists of supporting the respiration, prevention of hypotension, diuresis, hemodialysis, and in the event of phenobarbital poisoning, the administration of **sodium bicarbonate.** Tolerance does not develop to lethal doses.

Addiction

The abrupt withdrawal from barbiturates may cause tremors, restlessness, anxiety, weakness, nausea and vomiting, seizures, delirium, and cardiac arrest.

The Nonbarbiturates

The **benzodiazepine derivatives flurazepam** (Dalmane), **temazepam** (Restoril), and **triazolam** (Halcion) are all marketed as hypnotic agents.

VI

Diuretics and Cardiovascular Pharmacology

Cardiac Glycosides and Congestive Heart Failure

When the heart can no longer pump an adequate supply of blood to meet the metabolic needs of the tissues or in relation to venous return, cardiac failure may ensue.

A **compensatory mechanism** is brought into play in the event of **congestive heart failure:**

Cardiac dilatation and hypertrophy — taking advantage of the Frank-Starling relationship to utilize more contractile elements

Sympathetic stimulation — increasing the heart rate to maintain contractility and cardiac output

Increasing oxygen consumption through the arterial venous oxygen difference — increasing extraction of oxygen from limited blood flow

Production of aldosterone — increasing sodium and fluid retention, which may not be advantageous to the organism

Agents with **positive inotropic actions** that may be used in the management of congestive heart failure include the **cardiac glycosides** (e.g., digoxin and Digitoxin), **dopaminergic analogues** (e.g., dobutamine), **phosphodiesterase inhibitors** (e.g., amrinone and milrinone), **angiotensin antagonists** (e.g., captopril, enalapril, and lisinopril), and **vasodilators** (nitrates and hydralazine).

Cardiac Glycosides

The most important and often-used drugs in the treatment of congestive heart failure are the cardiac glycosides. ■ **Table 15-1** ■

Inotropic Action

Cardiac glycosides (digitalis) potentiate the coupling of electric excitation with mechanical contraction, and by augmenting the myoplasmic concentration of calcium, they provoke a more forceful contraction. It is thought that digitalis inhibits sodium-calcium exchanges by inhibiting Na^+K^+ ATPase. This results in

■ **Table 15-1** ■ Pharmacokinetic Profiles of Digoxin and Digitoxin

Properties	Digoxin	Digitoxin
Lipid solubility	Low	High
GI absorption	Good	Excellent
Protein binding	Low (25%)	High (90%)
Half-life	Short (1–2 d)	Long (6–9 d)
Enterohepatic recycling	Minimal	High
Liver metabolism	Low	High
Excretion	Active drug	Inactive metabolites
Onset of action after IV administration	Fast (5–30 min)	Slow (4–8 h)

an enhanced intracellular concentration of sodium, which in turn leads to a greater sodium influx that elicits stronger systolic contraction.

Modes of Action

The cardiac glycosides increase **cardiac output** through their positive inotropic effect. They slow **heart rate** by relieving the sympathetic tone and through their vagotonic effects. They reduce the **heart size** by relieving the Frank-Starling relationship. They increase **cardiac efficiency** by increasing cardiac output and decreasing oxygen consumption (decreased heart size and rate).

Blood pressure remains unchanged following the administration of cardiac glycosides. In **congestive heart failure,** the cardiac output is reduced, but the total peripheral resistance is increased, and these effects are reversed by cardiac glycosides.

Cardiac glycosides bring about **diuresis** by increasing both cardiac output and renal blood flow; the latter, in turn, reverses the **renal compensatory mechanism** activated in congestive heart failure. Consequently, the production of **aldosterone** is reduced, sodium retention is reversed, and the excretion of edematous fluid is enhanced. ■ **Fig. 15-1** ■

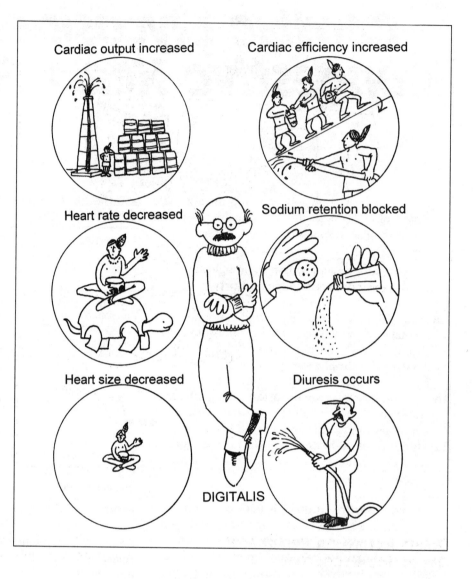

Cardiac output increased

Cardiac efficiency increased

Heart rate decreased

Sodium retention blocked

Heart size decreased

Diuresis occurs

DIGITALIS

■ Fig. 15-1 ■
Beneficial effects of
digitalis.

Digitalis Toxicity

The toxic effects of digitalis are frequent and may be fatal. Toxicity may result from **overdosage, decreased metabolism and excretion,** and **hypokalemia** stemming from the use of thiazide diuretics, diarrhea, and vomiting. Digitalis toxicity has several manifestations and includes any arrhythmia occurring de novo, renal insufficiency, electrolyte disturbances, visual symptoms, headache, psychotic symptoms, pulmonary disease, and anorexia.

Treatment of Digitalis Toxicity - Once digitalis toxicity is diagnosed, digitalis and diuretic use should be stopped. Furthermore, the patient should be monitored closely for any alteration in the pharmacokinetic profile of the cardiac glycoside being used. Treatment with **potassium** and magnesium may be indicated.

To manage digitalis-induced arrhythmia, **lidocaine,** with its fast onset and short duration of action is the drug of choice. **Phenytoin** may be used if potassium or lidocaine proves ineffective. **Propranolol** is effective in treating ventricular tachycardia. **Atropine** is effective if digitalis-induced conduction delay is at the atrioventricular node and is mediated via the vagus. Calcium channel-blocking agents such as **verapamil** are effective if the arrhythmia is due to reentry, increased diastolic depolarization in the Purkinje fibers, or oscillatory after-potential.

The antidigitoxin or the antidigoxin antibodies (**Digibind**) have been used to control digitalis intoxication. The antibody mobilizes depot digoxin and is excreted by the kidney as an antibody-digoxin complex.

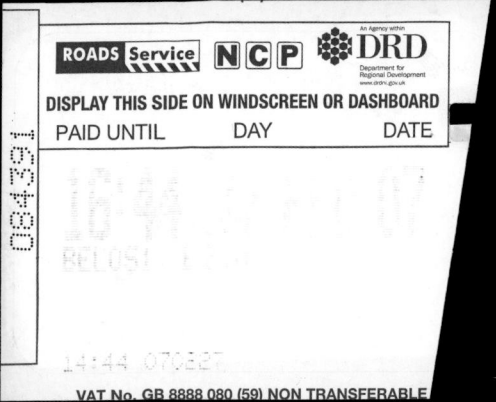

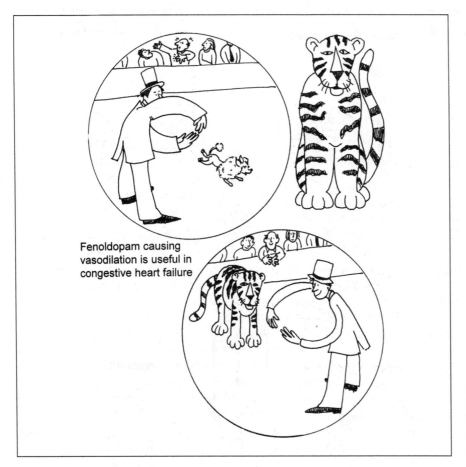

Fenoldopam causing vasodilation is useful in congestive heart failure

■Fig. 15-2 ■
Fenoldopam, which causes renal vasodilation, is an orally active dopamine$_1$-receptor agonist.

Drugs Acting on Peripheral Dopamine Receptors

Dobutamine, which is available only for parenteral administration, stimulates beta$_1$-adrenergic receptors, producing a strong inotropic effect.

Ibopamine, which is active orally, is capable of eliciting peripheral and renal vasodilation and a positive inotropic action. Ibopamine is converted to **epinine,** the active drug.

Fenoldopam is an orally active DA$_1$-receptor agonist. It is more potent than dopamine in causing renal vasodilation without having adrenergic, cholinergic, or histaminergic properties. **■ Fig. 15-2 ■**

Drugs Inhibiting Phosphodiesterase

Amrinone, milrinone, and **enoximone** exhibit a certain degree of selectivity for peak III phosphodiesterase, which is found predominantly in myocardial and vascular tissues. These agents exert positive inotropic and direct vasodilating actions.

Vasodilators and Angiotensin Antagonists

Nitrates and **hydralazine** have been used in patients with congestive heart failure.

An **angiotensin-converting enzyme** inhibitor such as **lisinopril** increases the left ventricular ejection fraction in patients with congestive heart failure. The drug's effectiveness is not diminished in the presence of impaired renal function.

In addition, a **vasodilator** in combination with an angiotensin-converting enzyme inhibitor has been used in congestive heart failure. The rationale for vasodilation in the management of congestive heart failure is based on the increased arteriolar vasotone that occurs. This initiates a vicious circle in which cardiac function is further depressed by an increase in afterload and in resistance to ejection.

Antiarrhythmic Drugs

Nature of Arrhythmias

Cardiac arrhythmias may be caused by a damaged heart, such as that produced by myocardial infarction, resulting from some abnormality in the blood supply to the pacemaker cells or conducting tissues, or both.

Arrythmias result from abnormalities in either **impulse generation** or **impulse conduction,** whereby the normal impulse conduction rate is slowed somewhere in the specialized conducting system of the heart. This disturbance is frequently, but not always, found in the atrioventricular node or in the bundles of His (heart block), or both.

The major electrophysiologic manifestations of impulse generation are found in the properties of **automaticity** (slope of phase 4 or diastolic depolarization) and of impulse conduction in **conduction velocity.** Drugs that alter pacemaker automaticity have a direct effect on the heart rate.

Rapid diastolic depolarization leads to a rapid rate of firing, whereas a lowered slope of phase 4 diastolic depolarization elicits fewer action potentials in the same time interval. Similarly, drugs that increase conduction velocity in the heart can help alleviate heart block, while those that decrease conduction velocity may slow a rapid heart rate.

Mechanism of Tachyarrhythmias

Tachyarrhythmias are generated by two mechanisms: **increased automaticity** or **reentry** due to the existence of a unidirectional block in a conducting system. Reentrant arrhythmias are abolished by:

- Increasing conduction velocity in abnormal tissue, thus removing the unidirectional block. **Phenytoin** and **lidocaine** can accomplish this.
- Decreasing conduction velocity in order to obtain bidirectional block. **Quinidine, procainamide,** and **propranolol** can achieve this.
- Increasing the refractory period relative to the action potential duration, so that the reentrant current becomes extinct in the refractory tissue. Most antiarrhythmic agents are able to do this.

Antiarrhythmic Agents

Antiarrhythmic agents ■ **Table 16-1** ■ are grouped according to the pattern of their electrophysiologic effects and their mechanisms of action. Antiarrythmic agents can cause **blockade of sodium channels** (quinidine, procainamide, disopyramide, moricizine, lidocaine, mexiletine, phenytoin, tocainide, encainide, flecainide, propafenone, and indecainide), **blockade of calcium channels** (verapamil and diltiazem), or **blockade of beta-adrenergic receptors** (propranolol, acebutolol, esmolol, and others), or they can **prolong repolarization** (amiodarone, bretylium, or sotalol). ■ **Fig. 16-1** ■

The **combination of various antiarrhythmic agents** in smaller doses is advocated. However, substances belonging to the same electrophysiologic class should not be combined, though drugs of different subsets of class I may be combined. Agents such as quinidine and amiodarone should not be given together because this combination may be associated with a considerable proarrhythmic effect. A combination of beta-adrenergic receptor blockers with class I antiarrhythmic drugs may be effective, mainly in patients whose arrhythmia is dependent on adrenergic stimulation. The combination of class III and IB substances can be useful in some cases from an electrophysiologic and clinical point of view. Among the **successful combinations** of this type are amiodarone and mexiletine, sotalol and mexiletine, and sotalol and tocainide.

Although many antiarrhythmic agents reduce automaticity, they may or may not reduce conduction velocity. ■ **Table 16-2** ■ See ■ **Table 16-1** ■

Pharmacology of Various Antiarrhythmic Agents

The pharmacology of some of the antiarrhythmic agents is summarized below and in ■ **Table 16-2** ■.

■ Table 16-1 ■ Antiarrhythmic Agents

Drugs	Recommended Dosage Regimens
Class IA	
Disopyramide	200–800 mg/day in 2 or 3 divided doses
Procainamide	750–6,000 mg/day in 3 or 4 divided doses
Quinidine	600–1,600 mg/day in 2–4 divided doses
Class IB	
Lidocaine	In adults, a loading dose of 150–200 mg administered over about 15 minutes; followed by a maintenance infusion of 2–4 mg/min to achieve a therapeutic plasma level of 2–6 μg/mL
Mexiletine	600–1,000 mg/day in 3 or 4 divided doses
Phenytoin	14 mg/kg loading dose, then 200–400 mg/day in 2 divided doses
Tocainide	800–1,800 mg/day in 2–4 divided doses
Class IC	
Encainide	75–200 mg/day in 3 or 4 divided doses
Flecainide	100–200 mg bid
Moricizine	Usual dosage: 200–300 mg, PO, tid
Propafenone	150–300 mg/8 h
Class II	
Acebutolol	400–1,200 mg/day in 2 divided doses
Esmolol	Available as a parenteral preparation containing 2.5 gm of drug in a 10-ml solution per ampule. For the treatment of supraventricular tachycardia, two ampules of esmolol are diluted in 500 ml of intravenous fluid to provide a solution of 10 mg of drug per milliliter.
Propranolol	40–240 mg/day in 3 or 4 divided doses
Class III	
Amiodarone	800–1,600 mg/day in divided doses for 5–14 days, then 200–800 mg/day for 5–14 days, then 100–400 mg/day thereafter
Bretylium	Available only for intravenous use. In adults, an intravenous bolus of bretylium tosylate, 5 mg/kg, administered over a 10-minute period. May be repeated after 30 minutes. Maintenance therapy: a similar bolus every 4–6 hours or by a constant infusion of 0.5–2 mg/min.
Class IV	
Verapamil	160–480 mg/day in divided doses
Others	
Digoxin	0.125–0.375 mg/day in a single dose
Encainide	75–200 mg/day in 3 or 4 divided doses
Flecainide	100–200 mg bid
Moricizine	Usual dosage: 200–300 mg, PO, tid
Propafenone	150–300 mg/8 h

Mexiletine

Mexiletine, which has a low first-pass metabolism, is used orally. It has a long half-life of 10–12 hours and is more effective than quinidine in treating ventricular couplets and ventricular tachycardia. It can cause tremor, ataxia, and nausea.

Tocainide

Like mexiletine, tocainide is a lidocaine analogue and has a long half-life of 10–15 hours. Tocainide causes hematologic abnormalities, including agranulocytosis, which is reversible.

Flecainide, Encainide, and Propafenone

Flecainide, encainide, and propafenone have a high affinity for sacrolemmal sodium channels. They are the most potent of the antiarrhythmic agents in slowing conduction of the cardiac impulse and in suppressing the intracellular sodium concentration and spontaneous ventricular premature complexes.

Beta-Adrenergic Antagonists

Propranolol, acebutolol, and esmolol are indicated for the treatment of arrhythmias. Metoprolol, propranolol, and timolol are used prophylactically after

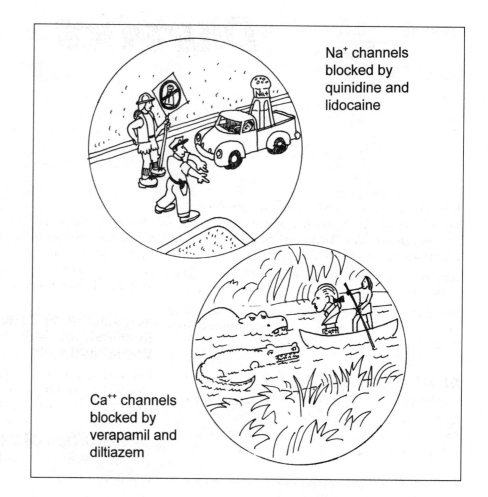

Na+ channels blocked by quinidine and lidocaine

Ca++ channels blocked by verapamil and diltiazem

■ Fig. 16-1 ■
Actions of antiarrhythmic agents.

■ Table 16-2 ■ Properties of Selected Antiarrhythmic Agents

Effects	Class IA: Quinidine, Procainamide	Class IA: Disopyramide	Class IB: Lidocaine, Phenytoin	Class II: Propranolol
Automaticity	↓	↓	↓	↓
Conduction velocity	↓	↓	0 or ↑	↓
Inotropism	(−)	(−)		(−)
Cardiac output	↓	↓	0 or ↓	
Blood pressure	↓	0 or ↓	0 or ↓	↓
Autonomic functions	Anticholinergic	Anticholinergic	−	Beta blockade

myocardial infarction to reduce the risk of sudden death in these patients.

Bretylium, Amiodarone, and Sotalol

Bretylium, amiodarone, and sotalol possess diverse pharmacologic properties. All share the capacity to prolong the duration of action potentials and the refractoriness that arises in Purkinje and ventricular muscle fibers.

Verapamil and Diltiazem

Verapamil and diltiazem are calcium channel blockers. The clinically important consequences of this action for the treatment of arrhythmias are the depression of calcium-dependent action potentials and the slowing of conduction in the atrioventricular node. Verapamil is the only calcium channel blocker that is currently marketed as an antiarrhythmic drug.

CHAPTER 17

Diuretics

The volume and composition of urine are controlled by the kidneys. The factors that govern these properties are **glomerular filtration, renal tubular resorption,** and **renal tubular secretion.**

The fractions of various substances filtered and resorbed in 24 hours are listed in ■ **Table 17-1** ■.

The distal tubule and collecting duct are permeable to water only in the presence of **antidiuretic hormone** (vasopressin).

Atrial Natriuretic Factor

Atrial natriuretic factor (ANF) is a polypeptide hormone that is secreted mainly by the heart atria in response to increases in atrial pressure or atrial stretch. ANF possesses the following characteristics:

- Modulates the glomerular filtration rate and excretion of fluids and electrolytes
- Modulates renal vascular resistance
- Decreases inner medullary hypertonicity and sodium resorption by tubular epithelial cells
- Stimulates sodium secretion in the inner medullary collecting duct cells; also modulates systemic vascular resistance, **inhibits the renin-angiotensin-aldosterone system,** and decreases arterial blood pressure, cardiac output, and plasma volume

Renal Dopaminergic (DA) Receptors, Diuresis, and Natriuresis

The DA_1 and DA_2 subtypes of dopamine receptors are localized in various regions within the kidney, including the renal vasculature (DA_1) as well as the sympathetic nerve terminals innervating the renal blood vessels (DA_2). Activation of these DA_1 receptors results in **natriuresis** and **diuresis.** In addition, dopamine can be synthesized within the proximal tubular lumen, and this locally produced dopamine plays an important role in regulating sodium excre-

tion, particularly during increases in sodium intake. The DA_1 receptor agonists such as **fenoldopam** (see ■ **Fig. 15-2** ■) can be beneficial in the treatment of hypertension, heart failure, and acute renal failure, and some selective DA_2 receptor agonists are also effective antihypertensive agents.

Regulation of Renal Sodium Channels by Aldosterone and Vasopressin

Aldosterone is considered the primary hormone responsible for regulating the resorption of sodium and secretion of potassium in the collecting duct.

Classification of Diuretics

The diuretics may be classified according to the following categories:

Carbonic anhydrase inhibitors
    Acetazolamide
    Dichlorphenamide
    Methazolamide
Loop diuretics
    Ethacrynic acid
    Bumetanide
    Furosemide
    Muzolimine
Thiazide diuretics
    Chlorothiazide
    Chlorthialidone
    Hydrochlorothiazide
    Metolazone
    Indapamide
Potassium-sparing diuretics
    Spironolactone
    Triamterene
    Amiloride
Osmotic diuretics
    Mannitol
    Urea

■ Table 17-1 ■ The Importance of Glomerulo-tubular Function in Fluid Volume Regulation

Substances Undergoing Glomerular Filtration	Percentage Resorbed
Sodium ion	99.4
Chloride ion	99.2
Bicarbonate ion	100.0
Urea	53.0
Glucose	100.0
Hydrogen ion	99.4
Potassium ion	100.0
Water	99.4

The major groups of diuretics and their sites of action are summarized in **■ Table 17-2 ■**.

Thiazide Diuretics

The thiazide diuretics vary in their actions. For instance, the potency of **hydrochlorothiazide** (HydroDIURIL and Esidrix) is ten times greater than that of **chlorothiazide** (Diuril), but the two drugs have equal efficacy.

They may cause **metabolic alkalosis** (resorption of bicarbonate and loss of hydrogen ions), **hyperuricemia** (enhanced resorption of uric acid), or **hyperglycemia** (inhibit insulin release directly and due to **hypokalemia**).

Use of Thiazide Diuretics

Edema - Thiazide diuretics are used in the treatment of edema of cardiac and GI origin and bring about a state of intravascular volume depletion.

Essential Hypertension - Thiazide diuretics are extremely effective in controlling essential hypertension. They exert their effects initially by bringing about volume depletion, then reduce the peripheral resistance and sensitivity of vascular receptor sites to catecholamines.

Idiopathic Hypercalciuria - The thiazides decrease the urinary calcium concentration by diminishing glomerular filtration and also enhance the urinary magnesium level.

Nephrogenic Diabetes Insipidus - The thiazide diuretics can reduce free water formation in patients with diabetes insipidus, in whom large amounts of free water are eliminated.

Loop Diuretics

The major loop diuretics are furosemide (Lasix) and ethacrynic acid (Edecrin). These agents inhibit the active resorption of chloride (and sodium) in the thick, ascending medullary portion of the loop of Henle and also in the cortical portion of the loop or the distal tubule. These agents are the most efficacious of the diuretics in the market, usually producing about a 20% loss in the filtered load of sodium (furosemide, 15–30%; ethacrynic acid, 17–23%).

Uses

Loop diuretics are used for treating the following conditions:

- Edema of **cardiac,** hepatic, or renal origin, including acute pulmonary edema and hypertensive crisis
- **Acute renal failure,** to maintain urine flow, though an excessive loss of extracellular fluid volume can cause a decrease in the glomerular filtration rate
- Hypercalcemia

Adverse Effects and Precautions

Excessive volume depletion, hyponatremia, and hypotension are major risks associated with the use of loop diuretics, and the side effects of **hypokalemia, hyperuricemia,** and **hyperglycemia** are always present. Loop diuretics should not be used concurrently with **ototoxic aminoglycoside antibiotics** (i.e., streptomycin, gentamicin, kanamycin, tobramycin).

Potassium-Sparing Diuretics

The potassium-sparing diuretics consist of **spironolactone** (Aldactone), which is an aldosterone antagonist, and **triamterene** (Dyrenium) and **amiloride** (Midamor), which exert their effects through a mechanism other than a mineralcorticoid action.

All act in the distal tubule, where the resorption of sodium is accompanied by the transfer of potassium into the lumen contents. When sodium resorption is hindered, potassium excretion is correspondingly reduced, such that more potassium is retained. The potassium-sparing diuretics are not very efficacious; they affect only 1–2% of the filtered load of sodium. All are given orally and eliminated in the urine, mostly by glomerular filtration, though some active tubular secretion may also occur.

Uses

A potassium-sparing diuretic can be given along with a thiazide or a loop diuretic to prevent hypokalemia. **Spironolactone** can also be beneficial in some pa-

■ Table 17-2 ■ Sites of Action of Diuretics

Drugs	Sites of Action
Sulfonamide diuretics Hydrochlorothiazide Chlorthalidone	Thick ascending limb (cortical) of the loop of Henle or distal tubule
Loop diuretics Furosemide Ethacrynic acid	Thick ascending limb (medullary) of the loop of Henle
Potassium-sparing diuretics Spironolactone (Aldactone) Triamterene Amiloride	Distal tubules
Uricosuric diuretics Tienilic acid	Thick ascending limb (cortical) of the loop of Henle
Osmotic diuretics Urea Mannitol	Proximal tubules, descending limb of the loop of Henle, and collecting tubule
Carbonic anhydrase inhibitors Acetazolamide Ethoxzolamide Dichlorphenamide	Proximal tubules

tients with severe congestive heart failure or cirrhosis associated with ascites.

Adverse Reactions and Cautions - The potassium-sparing diuretics should not be used concurrently with potassium supplements, as this combination is likely to produce **hyperkalemia**. Poor renal function also heightens the risk of hyperkalemia. Gastrointestinal disturbances, rash, drowsiness, and dizziness are all associated with their use. Spironolactone can cause the blood urea nitrogen level to increase and lead to menstrual irregularities.

CHAPTER 18

Vasodilators, Hypotensives, and Antihypertensive Medications

Blood Pressure and Its Control

Arterial blood pressure (BP) is proportional to the product of cardiac output (CO) multiplied by the peripheral vascular resistance (PVR):

$$BP = CO \times PVR$$

The anatomic sites responsible for maintaining blood pressure are the **heart,** the **kidney** (which regulates intravascular volume), the **arterioles,** and the **capacitance vessels.** The **baroreceptors,** which are modulated by sympathomimetic amines in conjunction with renin-directed angiotensin, also participate in maintaining normal blood pressure.

Antihypertensive medications reduce the activities of peripheral and central sympathetic systems, lower peripheral vascular resistance, interfere with renin-mediated **angiotensin** production, and promote sodium and volume depletion.

Classes of Antihypertensive Medication

The antihypertensive medications may be classified into the following groups:

Centrally acting hypotensive agents
    Clonidine
    Alpha-methyldopa
Alpha$_1$-adrenergic receptor antagonists
    Prazosin
Beta-adrenergic blocking agents
    Propranolol
    Metoprolol
Adrenergic neuron blockers
    Guanethidine

Arteriolar vasodilators
    Hydralazine
    Minoxidil
    Diazoxide
Arteriolar and venous dilators
    Sodium nitroprusside
Angiotensin-converting enzyme inhibitors
    Captopril
    Enalapril
    Lisinopril
Calcium channel antagonists
    Verapamil
    Nifedipine
    Diltiazem
    Nicardipine
Diuretics
    Thiazide(like) diuretics
    Potassium-sparing diuretics
    Loop diuretics

In clinical practice, the actual treatment of hypertension consists of a **stepped-care program,** which may involve the use of several drugs given sequentially in a predetermined regimen, which is modified on a regular basis as clinical judgment dictates.

Pharmacology of Antihypertensive Medications

Thiazide Diuretics

Besides being safe antihypertensive medications in themselves, the thiazide diuretics potentiate the effects of other medications used in controlling essential hypertension. Furthermore, many antihypertensive medications cause sodium and water retention, which can be reversed by diuretics.

Arteriolar and Venular Vasodilators

Hydralazine - Hydralazine (Apresoline) is the drug most often used in the treatment of **moderate to severe hypertension.** The decrease in total peripheral resistance it brings about causes reflex elevation of the heart rate and enhanced cardiac output. This cardiac acceleration, which may precipitate an **angina attack** in susceptible individuals, can be blocked with beta-adrenergic blocking agents.

Diazoxide - Diazoxide (Hyperstat), which is administered intravenously, is used exclusively in the management of **malignant hypertension** or a hypertensive crisis. It brings about reflex cardiac acceleration and increased cardiac output. However, it can cause hyperglycemia due to its inhibition of insulin release from the beta cells. Because diazoxide also produces sodium and water retention, it should be given with a diuretic such as furosemide or ethacrynic acid.

Minoxidil - Minoxidil (Loniten), which is effective orally, is indicated in patients with severe hypertension that has become refractory or has not responded to other drugs. The side effects of minoxidil include sodium retention, which can be controlled with a diuretic; tachycardia, which can be controlled with a beta blocker; and pronounced **hypertrichosis,** making it useful for the treatment of **alopecia.**

Nitroprusside - Nitroprusside (Nipride) is used exclusively in the management of **malignant hypertension** and a **hypertensive crisis.** Like diazoxide, nitroprusside is a vasodilator and has been used effectively in the care of patients with acute myocardial infarction and in patients with chronic refractory heart failure. Nitroprusside is given by infusion, and its blood pressure–lowering effect is directly related to the rate at which it is administered. When it is discontinued, blood pressure rises rapidly. Lethal **cyanide poisoning** may occur in patients with **rhodanase deficiency,** and thiocyanate may accumulate in patients with renal failure, thus inhibiting iodine uptake and causing hypothyroidism.

Prazosin - Prazosin (Minipress) is indicated in the treatment of **mild to severe hypertension.** It is a direct vasodilator and is used for long-term therapy. Its side effects are sedation, postural hypotension, and headache (due to vasodilation). As much as 97% of prazosin is bound to plasma protein. When used for the first time or in larger-than-recommended doses, prazosin may cause pronounced hypotension, faintness, dizziness, and palpitations. These effects, which have been labeled **first-dose phenomena,** are seen especially in salt- and water-depleted patients. Therefore, the initial dose of prazosin is small and is given at bedtime.

Adrenergic Neuronal Blocking Drugs

Guanethidine - Guanethidine (Ismelin) is the most potent drug for the management of **moderate to severe hypertension.** Its onset of action is slow. The effects of guanethidine on the adrenergic neurons include:

- A transient rise in blood pressure (resembles amphetamine and tyramine)
- Interference with neural conduction and neurally mediated catecholamine release (resembles bretylium)
- Catecholamine depletion (resembles reserpine)

Guanethidine abolishes sympathetic reflexes. As a result, postural hypotension occurs frequently with its use, as does **impotence.** In this regard, reserpine's effects are milder. The consequences of reduced sympathetic activity, such as diarrhea, bradycardia, and nasal stuffiness (cholinergic predominance), are observed with both reserpine and guanethidine. Unlike reserpine, guanethidine does not cross the blood-brain barrier and does not cause sedation and depression, while reserpine does. **Imipramine** blocks the antihypertensive effect of guanethidine.

Central Depressants of Sympathetic Functions

Alpha-Methyldopa - Alpha-methyldopa (Aldomet) is used for the control of **mild to severe hypertension.** It is converted to **alpha-methylnorepinephrine,** whose main hypotensive effect is due to stimulation of presynaptic alpha$_2$-adrenergic receptors, which leads to a reduction in the release of norepinephrine. In addition, it reduces the peripheral vascular resistance without altering the heart rate or cardiac output. Postural hypotension is mild and infrequent. Alpha-methyldopa can cause sedation, and tolerance to it can develop. **Coomb's test** will show up positive (25%) in patients who are taking the drug. Alpha-methyldopa has a long onset and a short duration of action. It is useful especially in the management of **hypertension complicated by renal dysfunction,** since it does not alter either renal blood flow or the glomerular filtration rate. It is contraindicated in patients with liver disease and may produce hepatitis-like symptoms.

Clonidine - Clonidine (Catapres) is used to treat mild to severe hypertension. Like alpha-methyldopa, it reduces sympathetic outflow centrally, has a vagotonic effect, and enhances sensitivity to carotid sinus stimulation. Heart rate and cardiac output are lowered. Abrupt withdrawal causes a rapid rise in blood pressure (**rebound hypertension**), which may require treatment with alpha- and beta-adrenergic blocking agents or even the reinstatement of clonidine itself.

Angiotensin-Converting Enzyme Inhibitors

Angiotensin II raises the blood pressure, and captopril reduces it according to the scheme in ■ **Fig. 18-1** ■.

Calcium Channel Antagonists

Verapamil, nifedipine, diltiazem, and **nicardipine** are used in the treatment of arrhythmias, ischemic heart disease, hypertrophic cardiomyopathy, and hypertension. ■ **Table 18-1** ■

■ **Table 18-1** ■ Comparison of the Hemodynamic Effects of Calcium Channel Antagonists

Effects	Nifedipine	Nicardipine	Verapamil
Vasodilation	+++	+++	++
Negative inotropic effect	0	0	++
Negative chronotropic effect	0	0	+++
Positive chronotropic effect*	+	+	0
Negative dromotropic effect (AV conduction)	0	0	+++
Cardiac output increases*	+	+	0

*Due to reflex stimulation.
AV = atrioventricular.

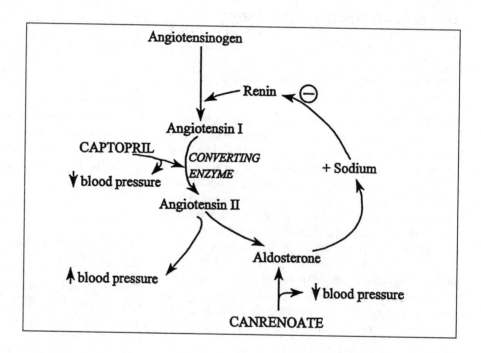

■ **Fig. 18-1** ■
The action of captopril.

CHAPTER 19

Antianginal Drugs

Angina pectoris is a sensation of strangulation, squeezing, and crushing of the chest.

Myocardial ischemia may lead to constant pain, which may be localized in the substernal area or become diffuse and radiate to the left shoulder and ulnar aspect of the left arm and hand. In addition, patients may experience anxiety, a feeling of impending death, shortness of breath, diaphoresis, nausea and vomiting, or syncope.

Oxygen Demand of the Heart

If the supply of oxygen to a portion of the heart is permanently deficient, necrosis develops, and a **myocardial infarction** takes place. If the oxygen deficiency is temporary, a painful coronary insufficiency, or **angina pectoris,** occurs.

The faster the heart beats, the more oxygen is needed, and the larger the heart is, the more oxygen is required for contraction. In addition, the greater the force of myocardial contraction is, the more oxygen is consumed. Agents effective in the management of angina pectoris accomplish their aim by **reducing oxygen demand,** not by increasing the oxygen supply. ■ **Fig. 19-1** ■

Nitrates and Nitrites

The mechanism underlying the therapeutic actions of nitrates and nitrites may be their ability to relax vascular smooth muscle and consequently **reduce cardiac preload** and **afterload.**

Cardiac Hemodynamics

The nitrates and nitrites bring about **arterial dilation,** and hence reduce blood pressure and the work of the heart. These agents also produce **venous dilation,** thereby decreasing the venous return and ventricular volume, which in turn diminishes wall tension. The end result of these events is a reduction in the work of the heart. By decreasing blood pressure, the heart rate is increased through the activation of carotid sinus reflexes. However, the extent of the reduction in wall tension is actually of greater benefit than the elevated heart rate. The nitrate-induced **tachycardia** may be blocked by the administration of **propranolol,** a beta-adrenergic receptor-blocking agent.

Coronary Circulation

Collateral vessels are silent blood vessels that become functional during hypoxic emergencies. By dilating, they permit greater blood flow to the ischemic areas, and nitrates accentuate this response.

Smooth Muscle

Nitrites and nitrates dilate blood vessels in all smooth muscles. When they dilate the cutaneous blood vessels, they cause blushing. When they dilate the cerebral vessels, they cause headache.

Pharmacokinetics

The nitrates and nitrites are best absorbed through the mucous membrane lining of the mouth and nose. Therefore they are usually administered sublingually or buccally.

Nonnitrate Coronary Vasodilators

Dipyridamole

Dipyridamole (Persantine) is used only as a prophylactic measure; it is not effective during an acute attack of angina. In contrast to nitroglycerin, dipyridamole dilates small resistance vessels (but not conducting or collateral vessels) by inhibiting the uptake and inactivation of **adenosine,** an effective coronary vasodilator. Dipyridamole also inhibits platelet aggregation.

Calcium Channel Entry Blockers

The calcium channel-blocking agents mediate their effects by decreasing myocardial contractility, de-

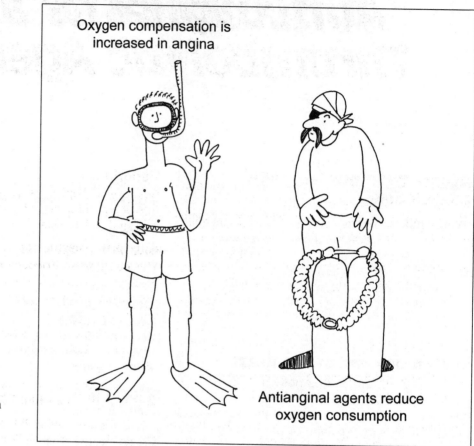

Oxygen compensation is
increased in angina

Antianginal agents reduce
oxygen consumption

■ **Fig. 19-1** ■
Oxygen consumption in
patients with angina
pectoris.

creasing heart rate, reducing the rate of conduction through the atrioventricular node, causing vasodilation, and reducing blood pressure.

Beta-Adrenergic Receptor-Blocking Agents

The beta-adrenergic receptor-blocking agents such as **propranolol** may be used prophylactically to pre-vent angina. By causing blockade of beta receptors in the heart, propranolol reduces blood pressure, cardiac contractility, cardiac output, and oxygen consumption. Because propranolol is a cardiac depressant, its injudicious use may lead to congestive heart failure. Propranolol is also frequently combined with nitrates to combat **nitrate-induced reflex tachycardia**.

CHAPTER 20

Anticoagulants and Thrombolytic Agents

Agents That Interfere with Coagulation

Therapeutic agents that interfere with blood coagulation fall into four classes:

1. **Anticoagulants,** which include heparin and the coumadin-inanedione oral anticoagulants
2. **Thrombolytic** agents, such as streptokinase, urokinase, and recombinant tissue-type plasminogen activator
3. **Antiplatelet** drugs, which alter the aggregating ability of platelets
4. **Defibrinogenating** agents, which remove the fibrinogen from circulating blood

Antithrombotic drugs are used clinically to prevent the formation of blood clots within the circulation (anticoagulant) or to dissolve a clot that has already formed (thrombolytic).

Heparin

Commercial heparin is a sulfated mucopolysaccharide of repeating units of D-glucosamine, D-glucuronic acid, and L-iduronic acid.

Oral Anticoagulants

The **coumarin anticoagulants** include dicumarol, warfarin sodium (coumadin sodium), warfarin potassium (Athrombin-K), acenocoumarol (Sintrom), and phenprocouman (Liquamar).

The **inanedione derivatives** are **phenindione** (Hedulin), **diphenadione** (Dipaxin), and **anisindione** (Miradon).

The comparative pharmacology of heparin and coumarin is shown in ■ **Table 20-1** ■.

The pharmacologic properties of oral anticoagulants are identical qualitatively, but their pharmacokinetic parameters and their toxicities vary. **Racemic warfarin sodium** is the most widely used anticoagulant.

■ Table 20-1 ■ Pharmacology of Heparin and Coumarin

Properties Studied	Heparin	Coumarin
Chemistry	High negative charge	
Occurrence	Naturally occurring in most tissues	Synthetic
Mechanism of action	Activates plasma antithrombin, blocks thromboplastin generation, neutralizes tissue thromboplastin	Inhibits the synthesis of factors II, VII, IX, and X by blocking the action of vitamin K
Pharmacokinetics		
Route of administration	Subcutaneously, intravenously	Orally
Onset	Minutes (10–20)	48 h
Duration	4 h (subcutaneously)	2–10 d
Protein binding and metabolism	In liver by heparinase; inactive metabolite is excreted by the kidney	Bound to albumin (99%), side-chain reduction to alcohol (dextrowarfarin), oxidation to 7-hydroxywarfarin (levowarfarin)
Antagonists	Protamine sulfate, strongly basic protein, forms complex with heparin to an inactive compound; 1 mg protamine for 100 units of heparin	Vitamin K, whole blood, fresh plasma

Cautions and Contraindications Concerning Anticoagulant Use

Bleeding

The use of anticoagulants is contraindicated in the presence of active hemorrhage, potential hemorrhage (acid pepsin disease), and hemorrhagic disorders (hemophilia).

Trauma

Anticoagulants should be used with extreme caution in patients with traumatic injuries to the CNS or the eyes because it is very difficult to control hemorrhage in these areas.

Pregnancy

Anticoagulant therapy during pregnancy is indicated for the treatment and prophylaxis of venous thromboembolic disease and systemic embolism associated with valvular heart disease or prosthetic heart valves. However, there are special problems that need to be considered when deciding on optimal anticoagulant therapy in pregnant women.

Heparin does not cross the placenta and is probably safe for the fetus. However, long-term heparin therapy is occasionally associated with maternal hemorrhage and rarely with symptomatic osteoporosis.

Coumarin derivatives cross the placenta and are potentially **teratogenic,** particularly in the first trimester. Neonatal hemorrhage is a risk if warfarin is administered to the pregnant mother near term.

Hypertension

The possible existence of an aneurysm must be considered in an untreated hypertensive patient.

Hepatic and Renal Failure and Other Conditions

Anticoagulant therapy should be monitored carefully in patients with severe hepatic or renal failure, vitamin K deficiency, or alcoholism and those with arthritis who are taking acetylsalicylic acid in large quantities. Furthermore, anticoagulants are extensively metabolized and their metabolites excreted, which can have an important bearing in patients suffering from renal disorders.

Drug-Drug Interactions

The incidence of interactions between the oral anticoagulants and other drugs, especially barbiturates, salicylates, and phenylbutazone, is numerous and at times may be life threatening. All aspects of the pharmacokinetics may be involved (see Chap. 1).

Various drugs can **augment the properties of oral anticoagulants** in a variety of ways:

- By displacing **extensively bound anticoagulants** from the plasma albumin (e.g., chloral hydrate, clofibrate, and phenylbutazone)
- By inhibiting **hepatic microsomal enzymes** (e.g., chloramphenicol and clofibrate)
- By reducing the **availability of vitamin K** (e.g., anabolic steroids and broad-spectrum antibiotics)
- By inhibiting **clotting factor synthesis** (e.g., anabolic steroids and salicylates)

There are also a number of agents that can **diminish the response to oral anticoagulants,** and they accomplish this by the following means:

- By inhibiting **absorption of anticoagulants** (e.g., griseofulvin and clofibrate)
- By inducing **hepatic microsomal enzymes** (e.g., barbiturates, ethchlorvynol, and glutethimide)
- By stimulating **clotting factor synthesis** (e.g., vitamin K)

These interactions have not been reported to occur with heparin.

Uses of Anticoagulants

Venous Thrombosis

An embolism may travel through the inferior vena cava, through the right heart, and eventually lodge in the lung, producing a **pulmonary embolism.** Susceptible patients may be treated prophylactically to diminish the risk of venous thrombosis.

Artificial Heart Valve

Foreign surfaces such as those introduced with artificial heart valves are more prone to be affected by clot formation. Although the introduction of newer techniques and materials for use in surgery has reduced the need for anticoagulants, they may be used effectively to prevent postoperative clot formation.

Atrial Fibrillation

In the presence of cardiac arrhythmias, when the heart is beating rapidly but inefficiently, the formation of clots in atrial appendages is common. When the heart is converting to a normal sinus rhythm, the clots may be freed and become lodged in vital organs. To avoid this, patients with arrhythmias may be treated with anticoagulants before and after conversion of the arrhythmia to a sinus rhythm.

Prophylaxis

Elderly individuals who have a sedentary lifestyle or patients confined to bed are more prone to thrombus formation. Other predisposing factors are reduced muscular mass and increased venous tortuosity. Anticoagulant therapy may be used in such patients to **lower the risk of thrombus formation**.

Certain Elective Surgical Procedures

In certain elective surgical procedures involving the lower legs and abdomen, heparin may be administered a few hours before surgery and continued for several days postoperatively.

Myocardial Infarction

Minidose heparin (1,500 units given subcutaneously) may be indicated in some but not all patients who have suffered a myocardial infarction.

Streptokinase (Streptase) is obtained from group C beta-hemolytic streptococci. **Urokinase** (Abbokinase) is obtained from urine. When these agents are used, the degradation of fibrin, fibrinogen, factors V and VII, and hemostatic plugs may precipitate hemorrhage, especially from sites of trauma and injury. Consequently, anticoagulants should not be used concomitantly with these agents. The effects of streptokinase or urokinase may be counteracted by **epsilon-aminocaproic acid.**

CHAPTER 21

Hematinics

Anemia is defined as a reduction in the circulating blood cell mass, which may be expressed as a reduction in the **volume of packed red blood cells** per deciliter, a reduction in the **blood hemoglobin concentration,** or a reduction in the **red blood cell count.**

Anemia can be caused by:

Ascorbic acid deficiency (anemia associated with scurvy)

Pyridoxine deficiency (vitamin B_6 is involved in the synthesis of delta-aminolevulinic acid, an intermediate in the biosynthesis of heme)

Riboflavin deficiency (glutathione reductase requires riboflavin)

Pantothenic acid deficiency (causes normocytic anemia)

Niacin deficiency (normocytic anemia)

Copper deficiency (copper is a cofactor for polyphenol oxidase, tyrosinase, cytochrome oxidase, lactase, and monoamine oxidase; in addition to ceruloplasmin, copper is also bound to erythrocuprein)

Zinc deficiency (carbonic anhydrase)

Chronic infection

Inflammation

Neoplastic disease

Erythropoietin

Erythropoietin is produced primarily by **peritubular cells** in the proximal tubule of the kidney.

Erythropoietin is effective for the treatment of anemia associated with **chronic renal failure.** It is also effective in managing the anemia seen in patients with **AIDS** who are being treated with **zidovudine** and the anemia associated with cancer chemotherapy.

Iron-Deficiency Anemia

The iron-deficiency anemias are caused by excessive loss or an inadequate intake of iron. In women, **men-**struation and **pregnancy** may increase the iron requirement. Iron deficiency in men, as well as women, may be due to blood loss resulting from hemorrhage associated with gastric ulcer or neoplasm. In children, iron deficiency is due to a nutritionally inadequate diet.

Metabolism of Iron

Iron is absorbed better in **ferrous** (Fe^{2+}) than in the **ferric** (Fe^{3+}) form. The extent of **absorption of iron** from the duodenum is thought to be regulated by mucosal proteins, and a process referred to as *mucosal block.* The absorbed iron is either stored in mucosal **ferritin** or transported to plasma and bound to **transferrin.** Ferrous calcium citrate is most used in patients during pregnancy to provide iron as well as calcium.

Iron Toxicity

The initial signs and symptoms of iron poisoning are GI and usually consist of nausea, vomiting, and diarrhea. If toxicity is untreated, acidosis, cyanosis, and circulatory collapse may ensue. Treatment should include induced vomiting and lavage if the poisoning is discovered early, catharsis to hasten evacuation, sodium bicarbonate therapy to combat the acidosis, and the administration of **deferoxamine** (Desferal), a specific iron-chelating agent.

Megaloblastic Anemias, Folic Acid, and Vitamin B₁₂

Both **vitamin B_{12}** and **folic acid** are essential for the synthesis of DNA, and this process is impaired in patients with megaloblastic anemia. **Vitamin B_{12} deficiency** may result from many factors, including:

- Failure of secretion of the glycoprotein intrinsic factor of Castle (pernicious anemia)
- Absence of intestinal receptors for the intrinsic factor

- Gastrectomy (achlorhydria and lack of intrinsic factor)
- Malabsorption syndrome (idiopathic steatorrhea)
- Intestinal parasites (fish tapeworms)
- Lack of vitamin B_{12}-binding protein in plasma (transcobalamin II and alpha and beta globulin)
- Vitamin B_{12} antagonist (antibody to intrinsic factor)

Vitamin B_{12} must be administered parenterally.

Folic acid deficiency may result from:

- Nutritional deficiency
- Malabsorption syndrome
- Reduced folate-binding protein
- Folic acid antagonists (e.g., **methotrexate**)
- Drugs reducing the level of folic acid (**anticonvulsants** and **pyrimethamine**)
- Agents blocking purine synthesis (e.g., **mercaptopurine, thioguanine**) or pyrimidine synthesis (**5-fluorouracil**)
- Hemolytic diseases (accelerated hematopoiesis)
- Prolif erative diseases and other conditions

Folic acid is administered orally and should not be used in the treatment of pernicious anemia.

CHAPTER 22

Treatment of Hyperlipoproteinemias

Synthesis of Cholesterol

Cholesterol, which is essential for the synthesis of adrenal, ovarian, and testicular steroid hormones, originates from two sources. The body synthesizes approximately 2 g of cholesterol per day. In addition, between 300 and 800 mg of cholesterol is ingested a day, depending on a person's diet. Between 300 and 1,500 mg of cholesterol is excreted per day.

Therapy for Lipoprotein Abnormalities

The treatment of **hyperlipoid state** may include reducing the intake of cholesterol, increasing the excretion of cholesterol, or reducing the synthesis of cholesterol.

Competitive Inhibitors of HMG-CoA Reductase

These reductase inhibitors are structural analogues of 3-hydroxy-3-methylglutaryl-coenzyme A (HMG-CoA). The first drug in this class was compactin. A close congener, **lovastatin,** is widely used. **Simvastatin, pravastatin,** and **fluvastatin** are similar drugs.

Clofibrate - Clofibrate (Atromid S) reduces very low density lipoprotein (VLDL), triglyceride, and cholesterol levels. Clofibrate increases extrahepatic lipoprotein lipase activity but not hepatic lipase activity. Thus the triglyceride-lowering effect of clofibrate may be caused by increased efficiency of removal of VLDL, as well as by reduced VLDL secretion by the liver. Because clofibrate displaces **coumarin** and **phenytoin** from binding sites, the **prothrombin time** should be checked on a regular basis in patients who are taking both agents. A flulike syndrome, characterized by muscular cramps, tenderness, stiffness, and weakness, may occur in some patients.

Cholestyramine

Cholestyramine (Questran) is not absorbed but binds to bile acids in the intestine and then is eliminated.

To replenish the lost bile acid, cholesterol is converted to bile acid, and this lowers the level of cholesterol. Cholestyramine has also been used in the treatment of **cholestasis** to control intense pruritis.

Besides binding to bile acid, cholestyramine binds to numerous drugs used in the management of cardiovascular diseases, which may be taken along with cholestyramine. These include chlorthiazide, phenylbutazone, phenobarbital, anticoagulants, digitalis, and fat-soluble vitamins (A, D, E, and K). Consequently, these and similar agents should be taken 1 hour before or 4 hours after the administration of cholestyramine.

Nicotinic Acid

Nicotinic acid inhibits the release of free fatty acids, followed by a fall in the VLDL and then the low-density lipoprotein (LDL) level. Nicotinic acid may cause intense flushing and itching (histamine release and vasodilation), and tolerance develops to this effect.

Thyroxine

Hypothyroidism is associated with elevated levels of plasma lipids, and the reverse is the case with hyperthyroidism. D-thyroxine (Choloxin) increases the synthesis of cholesterol in the liver but increases the fecal excretion of cholesterol and the rate of conversion of cholesterol to bile acid. Consequently, the level of LDL is reduced. The recommended dose of D-thyroxine is 2–6 mg; in higher than therapeutic doses, it may produce nervousness or insomnia, cause cardiac dysrhythmias, or precipitate an anginal attack.

Probucol

Probucol (Lorelco) lowers the cholesterol level, and hence the LDL level, after 1–3 months of treatment. Therefore, it is indicated in the management of type II hyperlipoproteinemia. The few side effects reported for probucol use are transient flatulence and diarrhea.

VII

Endocrine Pharmacology

CHAPTER 23

Antidiabetic Agents

Diabetes mellitus results from disturbances in the metabolism of carbohydrates, lipids, and proteins.

The **release of insulin** is closely coupled with the glucose level. **Hypoglycemia** results in a low level of **insulin** and a high level of **glucagon,** and hence favors the processes of **glycogenolysis** and **gluconeogenesis.** ■ **Fig. 23-1** ■

Growth hormone is one of glucose's counterregulatory hormones. It is released in response to hypoglycemia and has intrinsic hyperglycemic actions as well as causes insulin resistance.

Classes of Diabetes Mellitus

There are two types of diabetes mellitus: type I, or **insulin-dependent diabetes mellitus,** and type II, or **non-insulin-dependent diabetes mellitus.** Type I diabetic patients are dependent on insulin to prevent

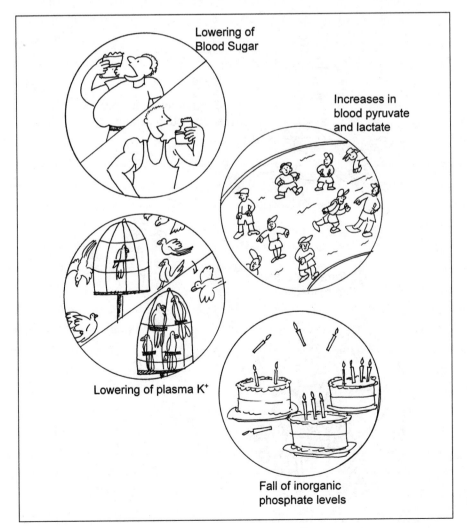

Lowering of Blood Sugar

Increases in blood pyruvate and lactate

Lowering of plasma K⁺

Fall of inorganic phosphate levels

■ **Fig. 23-1** ■
Modes of action of insulin.

ketosis and have insulinopenia. Type II diabetic patients, who are non-insulin-dependent, are not prone to ketosis.

The Insulin Receptor

When insulin binds to specific membrane receptors on target cells, this initiates a wide spectrum of biologic activities. It:

- Enhances the transport of sugar and amino acids
- Stimulates anabolic pathways
- Stimulates growth and development by triggering RNA and DNA synthesis

The **insulin receptor** is a **disulfide-linked oigomer** consisting of two alpha and two beta chains. The insulin receptor is internalized, and this action terminates the insulin signal at the surface of the cell. Once internalized, some of the receptors are degraded, and others are recycled back to the membrane. In addition, phosphatases are able to dephosphorylate the phosphorylated insulin receptor. This dephosphorylation reduces kinase activity and decreases the responsiveness to insulin.

Treatment of Diabetes Mellitus

Drug Treatment

The drug treatment of diabetes mellitus includes eliminating **obesity** (which causes resistance to both endogenous and exogenous forms of insulin), **exercising** (to promote glucose utilization and reduce insulin requirement), **dieting** (to restrict intake of excess amounts of carbohydrates), and **taking insulin** (primarily in polyuric, polydipsic, and ketonuric patients).

Insulin - *Insulin preparations* are fast, intermediate, or long acting. ■ **Fig. 23-2** ■

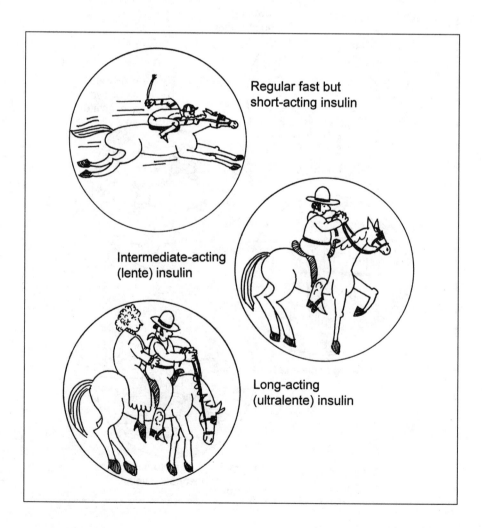

Regular fast but short-acting insulin

Intermediate-acting (lente) insulin

Long-acting (ultralente) insulin

■ **Fig. 23-2** ■
Various insulin preparations.

Crystalline (regular) **insulin** may be used as a supplemental injection or for instituting corrective measures in the management of infection and trauma, for postoperative stabilization, and for the rehabilitation of patients recovering from ketoacidosis and coma. In addition, neutral protamine Hagedorn contains regular insulin.

Ultralente or **semilente insulin** is used to eliminate nocturnal and early morning hyperglycemia.

COMPLICATIONS OF INSULIN THERAPY - **Hypoglycemia,** a primary complication of insulin therapy, may result from an excess of insulin or a lack of glucose, or both. Severe hypoglycemia may cause headache, confusion, double vision, drowsiness, and convulsions. The treatment of this hypoglycemia may include the administration of glucose or glucagon.

Lipodystrophy can also result from insulin therapy and is characterized by atrophy of subcutaneous fat. **Insulin edema** is manifested by a generalized retention of fluid. **Insulin resistance** arises when there is an excess insulin requirement that exceeds 200 units/day. ■ **Fig. 23-3** ■

AGENTS THAT ALTER THE RELEASE OF INSULIN - The release of insulin is enhanced by certain physiologic substances (glucose, leucine, arginine, gastrin, secretin, and pancreozymin) and by certain pharmacologic agents (oral hypoglycemic agents). ■ **Fig. 23-4** ■

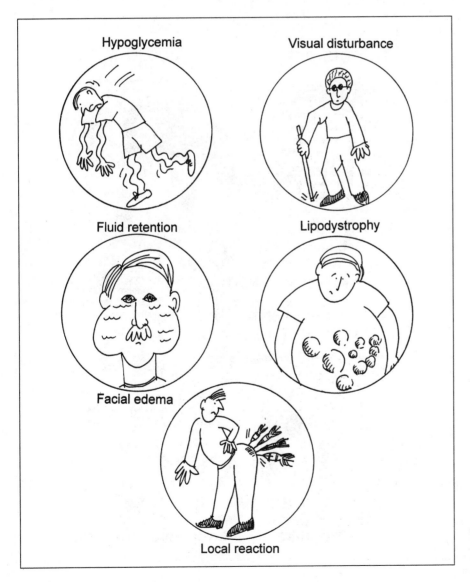

Hypoglycemia

Visual disturbance

Fluid retention

Lipodystrophy

Facial edema

Local reaction

■ **Fig. 23-3** ■
Adverse effects of insulin therapy.

The release of insulin is also inhibited by some physiologic substances (epinephrine and norepinephrine) as well as by some pharmacologic substances (thiazide diuretics, diazoxide, and chlorpromazine).

Oral Hypoglycemic Agents - Oral hypoglycemic agents have advantages over insulin, because, by releasing insulin and by decreasing the release of glucagon, they mimic physiologic processes and cause fewer allergic reactions. See ■ **Fig. 23-4** ■

The mechanisms that underlie the hypoglycemic actions of **sulfonylureas** are:

Pancreatic
Improved insulin secretion
Reduced glucagon secretion

Extrapancreatic
Improved tissue sensitivity to insulin
   Direct
   Increased receptor binding
   Improved post-binding action
   Indirect
   Reduced hyperglycemia
   Decreased plasma free fatty-acid
     concentrations
   Reduced hepatic insulin extraction

RECEPTORS FOR SULFONYLUREA AND THEIR MECHANISM OF ACTION - Sulfonylureas such as **glyburide** and **glipizide** bind to sulfonylurea receptors located on the surface of beta cells and trigger insulin releases at nanomolar concentrations. Sulfo-

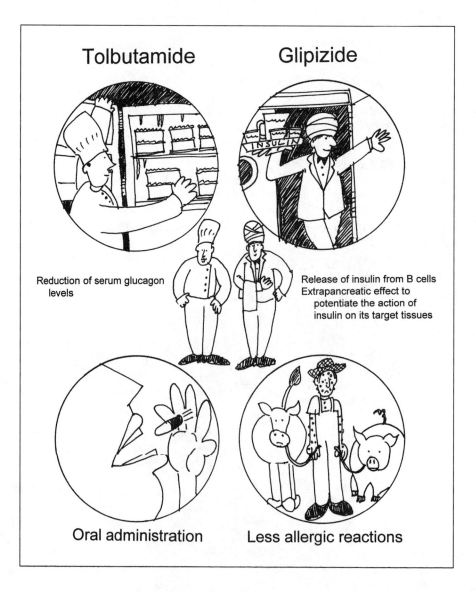

Tolbutamide   **Glipizide**

Reduction of serum glucagon levels

Release of insulin from B cells
Extrapancreatic effect to potentiate the action of insulin on its target tissues

Oral administration   Less allergic reactions

■ **Fig. 23-4** ■
Oral hypoglycemic agents.

nylureas bind to ATP-sensitive potassium channels and inhibit potassium efflux through these channels. The inhibition of ATP-sensitive potassium channels then leads to depolarization of the beta cells; this opens voltage-dependent calcium channels and allows the entry of extracellular calcium. The rising level of cytosolic-free calcium next triggers the release of insulin. An increase in the cyclic adenosine monophosphate levels in the cells can also open the voltage-dependent calcium channels, thus increasing calcium influx into the cells.

Treatment of Diabetic Ketoacidosis

Diabetic ketoacidosis may result from or be aggravated by infection, surgery, trauma, shock, emotional stress, or failure to take sufficient amounts of insulin. Treatment is focused on reversing the **hypokalemia** by administering potassium chloride and on offsetting the **acidosis** by providing bicarbonate. The **dehydration** and **electrolyte imbalance** are treated with appropriate measures, and crystalline zinc insulin is administered to counter the **hyperglycemia.**

CHAPTER 24

Adrenal Steroids

The **adrenal gland,** located at the cap of the kidney, is divided histologically into three zones: the outer zone or **zona glomerulosa,** the middle zone or **zona fasciculata,** and the inner zone or **zona reticularis.** The adrenal cortex synthesizes **cholesterol** and **pregnenolone** through the interaction of a group of enzymatic reactions.

Classification of Adrenal Steroids

The adrenal steroids are divided into three major categories: **glucocorticoids, mineralocorticoids,** and **sex hormones.**

The Glucocorticoids

The glucocorticoids mainly influence carbohydrate metabolism and, to a certain extent, protein and lipid metabolism. The main glucocorticoid is **cortisol,** with a daily secretion of 15 mg. Cortisol, corticosterone, aldosterone, and the synthetic steroids used in steroid therapy (e.g., prednisolone, dexamethasone, and triamcinolone) are **glucocorticoid agonists** and therefore elicit glucocorticoid responses. ■ **Fig. 24-1** ■

A number of other steroids bind to the glucocorticoid receptor and thus suppress glucocorticoid responses.

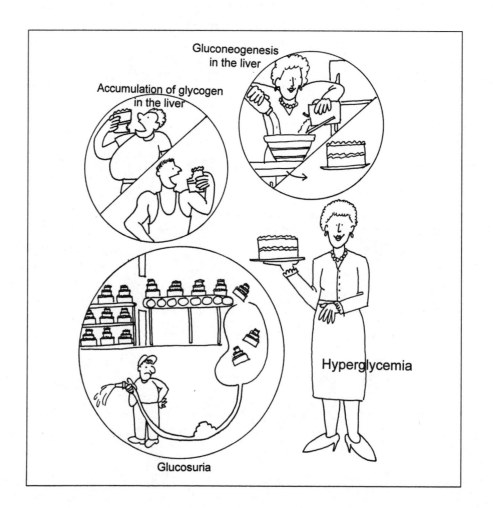

Gluconeogenesis in the liver

Accumulation of glycogen in the liver

Hyperglycemia

Glucosuria

■ **Fig. 24-1** ■
Metabolic actions of corticosteroids.

The Mineralocorticoids

The mineralocorticoids influence **salt** and **water metabolism** and in general conserve sodium levels. They promote the resorption of sodium and the secretion of potassium in the cortical collecting tubules and possibly the connecting segment. They also elicit hydrogen secretion in the medullary collecting tubules. ■ **Fig. 24-2 and Fig. 24-3** ■

The main mineralocorticoid is **aldosterone,** with a daily secretion of 100 μg. Aldosterone is synthesized from 18-hydroxy-corticosterone by a dehydrogenase. The consequence of 18-hydroxy-corticosterone dehydrogenase deficiency is diminished secretion of aldosterone; the clinical manifestations are sodium depletion, dehydration, hypotension, potassium retention, and enhanced plasma renin levels.

Sex Hormones

Small quantities of **progesterone, testosterone,** and **estradiol** are also produced by the adrenal gland.

Actions and Pharmacologic Applications of Glucocorticoids

The glucocorticoids possess a plethora of physiologic actions, including a role in **differentiation** and **development.** They are vital in the treatment of adrenal insufficiency and are used extensively in large pharmacologic doses as antiinflammatory and immunosuppressive agents. ■ **Fig. 24-4** ■ Some of the nonendocrine conditions for which they may be used are arthritis, tenosynovitis, systemic lupus erythematosus, acute rheumatic carditis, bronchial asthma,

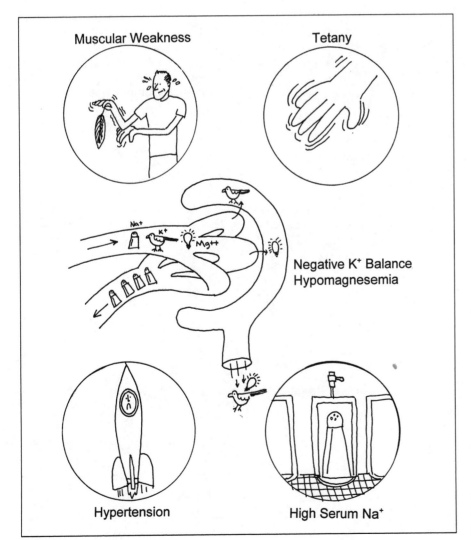

Muscular Weakness

Tetany

Negative K$^+$ Balance
Hypomagnesemia

Hypertension

High Serum Na$^+$

■ **Fig. 24-2** ■
Nature of primary aldosteronism.

organ transplantation, ulcerative colitis, cerebral edema, and myasthenia gravis.

Glucose Metabolism

Cortisol has an antiinsulin effect and aggravates the pathologic consequences of diabetes mellitus. It increases gluconeogenesis, inhibits the peripheral utilization of glucose, and causes hyperglycemia and glucosuria. ■ **Fig. 24-5** ■ See ■ **Fig. 24-1** ■

Protein Metabolism

Cortisol promotes the breakdown of proteins and inhibits protein synthesis. ■ **Fig. 24-6** ■ This leads to muscle wasting in the quadriceps-femoris groups, and muscular activities may become difficult as a result. The effect of cortisol is opposite to that of insulin.

Glycogen Metabolism

The effects of glucocorticoids on glycogen accumulation appear to be predominantly, although not exclusively, insulin dependent, since glycogen accumulation is markedly reduced in pancreatectomized animals. Glucocorticoid-stimulated increases in insulin secretion promote further glycogen accumulation. See ■ **Fig. 24-1** ■

Lipid Metabolism

Cortisol causes the abnormal deposition of a fat pad called "buffalo hump." See ■ **Fig. 24-6** ■

■ **Fig. 24-3** ■
Nature of secondary aldosteronism.

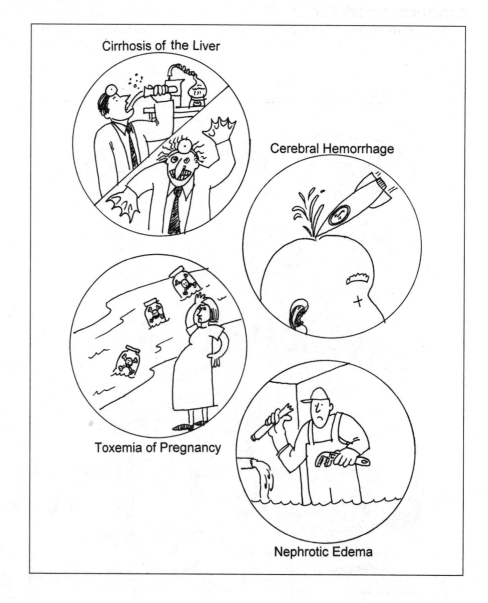

Electrolytes and Water Metabolism

Cortisol use can bring about hypernatremia, hypokalemia, and hypercalciuria.

Uric Acid

Cortisol use causes hyperuricemia by suppressing the renal tubular resorption of uric acid.

Gastric Hydrochloric Acid

Cortisol promotes the production of gastric hydrochloric acid. See ■ Fig. 24-5 ■

Blood Coagulation

Cortisol, like epinephrine, augments the coagulability of blood.

Antiinflammatory Action

Cortisol exerts its antiinflammatory effect in part by blocking the release and action of histamine. See ■ Fig. 24-4 ■ In addition, it decreases the migration of polymorphonuclear leukocytes.

Hematologic Effects

Cortisol produces eosinophilia and causes the involution of lymphoid tissues.

Leukocytes

The administration of glucocorticoids to human subjects brings about lymphocytopenia, monocytopenia, and eosinopenia. In addition, glucocorticoids block a number of lymphocytic functions.

Immunosuppression

Although considered to be immunosuppressive, therapeutic doses of glucocorticoids do not significantly decrease the concentration of antibodies in the circulation. Furthermore, during glucocorticoid therapy, patients exhibit a nearly normal antibody response to antigenic challenge.

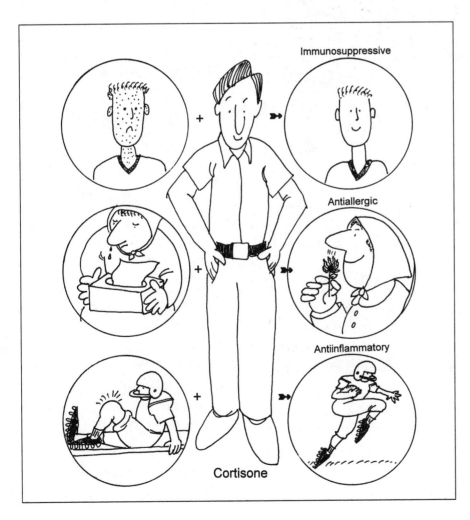

■ Fig. 24-4 ■
Therapeutic usefulness of corticosteroids.

Central Nervous System Effects

Glucocorticoids, which penetrate the blood-brain barrier, affect behavior, mood, and neural activity, and they are able to regulate the permeability of the blood-brain barrier to other substances. Hence they are used to treat brain edema.

Calcium Metabolism

Glucocorticoids are used to treat certain hypercalcemias — largely granulomatous conditions such as **sarcoidosis** in which the steroid blocks the forma-tion of 1-alpha,25-dihydroxycholecalciferol by the granulomatous tissues.

Contraindications to Glucocorticoid Therapy

Besides the adverse effects just described, glucocorticoid therapy is contraindicated under the following circumstances: diabetes mellitus, digitalis therapy, glaucoma, hypertension, osteoporosis, peptic ulcer, tuberculosis, and viral infection. See ▪ **Fig. 24-5** ▪

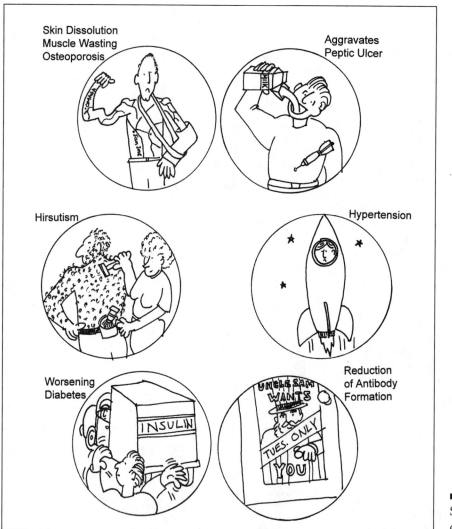

▪ **Fig. 24-5** ▪
Side effects of corticosteroids.

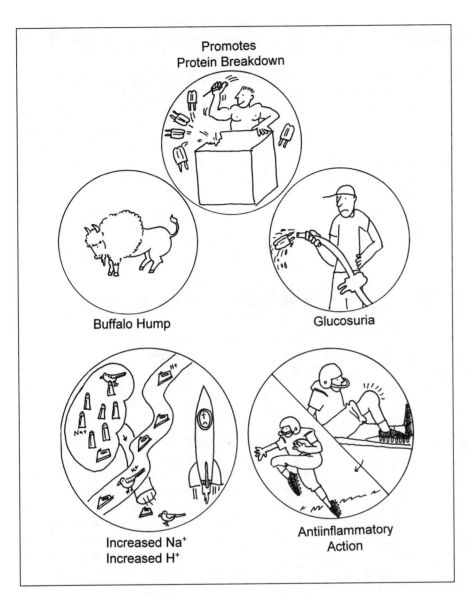

■ Fig. 24-6 ■
Pharmacologic actions of corticosteroids.

CHAPTER 25

Thyroid Hormones and Their Antagonists

The **thyroid gland** synthesizes **thyroxine** (T_4) and **triiodothyronine** (T_3). These hormones are involved in the regulation of

- Growth and development
- Thermoregulation and calorigenesis
- Metabolism of carbohydrates, proteins, and lipids
- Hypophyseal thyrotropin secretion ■ **Fig. 25-1** ■

The thyroid gland also synthesizes **calcitonin,** which produces hypocalcemia by inhibiting bone resorption and by enhancing the urinary excretion of calcium and phosphate.

Synthesis of Thyroid Hormones

The steps involved in the synthesis of thyroid hormones are depicted in ■ **Fig. 25-2** ■ . First, the ingested iodide (100–150 μg/day) is actively transported (**iodide trapping**) and then accumulated in the thyroid gland. Following this, the trapped iodide is oxidized by a peroxidase system to active iodine, which iodinates the tyrosine residue of glycoprotein to yield **monoiodotyrosine** (MIT) and **diiodotyrosine** (DIT). This process is called **iodide organification.** The MIT and DIT combine to form T_3, whereas two molecules of DIT combine to form T_4. T_3 and T_4 are released from thyroglobulin through the actions of pinocytosis and the proteolysis of thyroglobulin by lysosomal enzymes. In the circulation, 75% of T_4 is bound to **thyroxine-binding globulin** (TBG), and the remainder is mostly bound to **thyroxine-binding prealbumin** (TBPA). Approximately 0.05% of T_4 remains free. T_3 is similarly bound to TBG, allowing only 0.5% of it to remain in the free form. See ■ **Fig. 25-2** ■

Catabolism of T_4

T_4 may undergo deamination, decarboxylation, and glucuronic acid conjugation. However, it is deiodi-

nated in one of two ways: it may be deiodinated to 3, 5,3′-triiodothyronine, which is more efficacious than T_4, or it may be deiodinated to the pharmacologically inactive 3,3′5-triiodothyronine (**reverse T_3**).

Regulation of Thyroid Hormone Production

The production of thyroid hormones is regulated in two ways: (1) by **thyrotropin** and (2) by a variety of nutritional, hormonal, and illness-related factors. The secretion of thyrotropin is regulated by the circulating levels of T_4 and by thyrotropin-releasing hormone (TRH). ■ **Fig. 25-3** ■

The Action of Thyrotropin

Thyrotropin is synthesized by **thyrotrophs** located in the anterior pituitary gland and consists of two peptide subunits: the **alpha subunit** (seen also in luteinizing hormone, follicle-stimulating hormone, and chorionic gonadotropin) and the **beta-subunit,** which determines the biologic activities of thyrotrophs. T_3 and T_4 inhibit both the synthesis and release of thyrotropin. See ■ **Fig. 25-3** ■

Hypothalamic Pituitary-Thyroid Interaction

The concentration of thyroid-stimulating hormone (TSH) increases rapidly following the administration of TRH. In hyperthyroidism, the high levels of T_3 and T_4 inhibit the action of TSH and cause a lack of response to TRH. See ■ **Fig. 25-3** ■

Treatment of Hyperthyroidism

The treatment for hyperthyroidism includes the following:

- Treating the cause of the hyperthyroidism
- Antithyroid therapy
- Drugs: Propylthiouracil, methimazole, iodide, or iodine 131

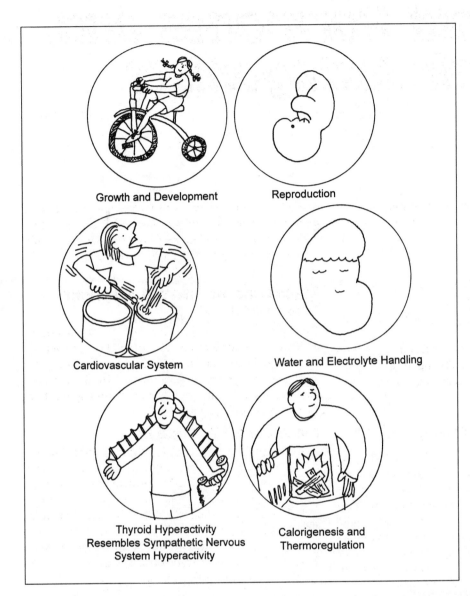

Growth and Development

Reproduction

Cardiovascular System

Water and Electrolyte Handling

Thyroid Hyperactivity
Resembles Sympathetic Nervous
System Hyperactivity

Calorigenesis and
Thermoregulation

■ **Fig. 25-1** ■
Actions of thyroid hormones.

- Subtotal thyroidectomy
- Inhibition of peripheral T_3 production with propylthiouracil, sodium ipodate and iopanoic acid, or glucocorticoids
- Amelioration of thyroid hormone action using propranolol and similar drugs

Agents That Inhibit Iodide Trapping

Monovalent anions such as **perchlorate** (ClO_4^-), **pertechnetate** (TCO_4^-), and **thiocyanate** (SCN^-) competitively inhibit the active transport and accumulation of iodide. The effect is reversible with large concentrations of iodide. However, these agents are now obsolete and no longer used. **Goitrogenic vegetables** such as cabbage contain thiocyanate.

Agents That Inhibit the Synthesis of Thyroid Hormones

Propylthiouracil, methimazole, and **carbimazole** exert their effects by inhibiting **iodide organification** and by inhibiting the **formation of DIT.** These agents all possess a thiocarbamide moiety ($-N-\overset{\overset{S}{\|}}{C}-R$) which is essential for their antithyroid actions. The onset of their beneficial effects is slow and takes 3–4 weeks.

Agents That Inhibit Thyroid Hormone Release

Iodides such as potassium iodide and **Lugol's solution,** which contain 5% iodine and 10% potassium iodide, exert their beneficial effects by inhibiting or-

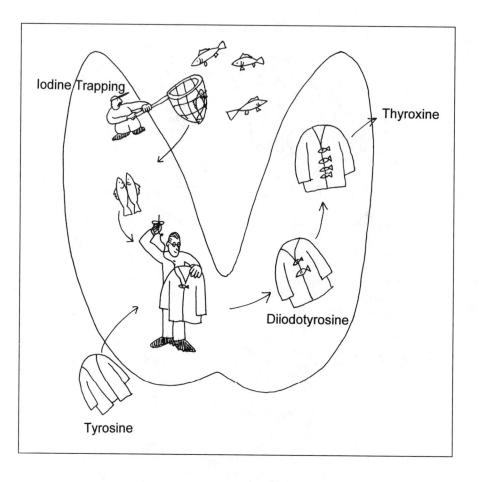

■ Fig. 25-2 ■
Synthesis of thyroxine.

ganification, inhibiting the release of thyroid hormones, and decreasing (inhibiting proteolysis) the size and vascularity of the gland. This makes them useful for preparing the patient for surgery.

Treatment of Thyrotoxicosis

Iodine 131 is given orally in **older patients** for the treatment of thyrotoxicosis. It accumulates in the storage follicles and emits beta rays with a half-life of 5 days. Radioactive iodine, which crosses the placental barrier, is contraindicated in pregnant women.

The major complication following either surgery or treatment with radioactive iodine may be **hypothyroidism,** which requires replacement therapy with **levothyroxine.**

Treatment of Thyrotoxic Crisis

The synthesis of thyroid hormone should be inhibited by using a large dose of propylthiouracil (200 mg q4h). Propylthiouracil also inhibits the conversion of T_4 to T_3.

The release of thyroid hormone may be inhibited by sodium iodide given intravenously.

Large doses of dexamethasone should be given orally. This steroid inhibits the release of thyroid hormone and the conversion of T_4 to T_3.

Large doses of adrenergic antagonists such as propranolol, reserpine, or guanethidine may be tried.

Digitalis and diuretics may be required in the event of congestive heart failure.

Antipyretics should be administered to reduce fever.

Any other supportive measures should be instituted to reduce the high risk of death.

Treatment of Hypothyroidism

Levothyroxine (Levothroid and Synthroid; 2–25 μg/kg) is given for replacement therapy in patients with hypothyroidism. Following are other **thyroid preparations:**

Thyroglobulin (Proloid) is purified from hog thyroid gland and standardized to yield a T_4 to T_3 ratio of 2.5 to 1.

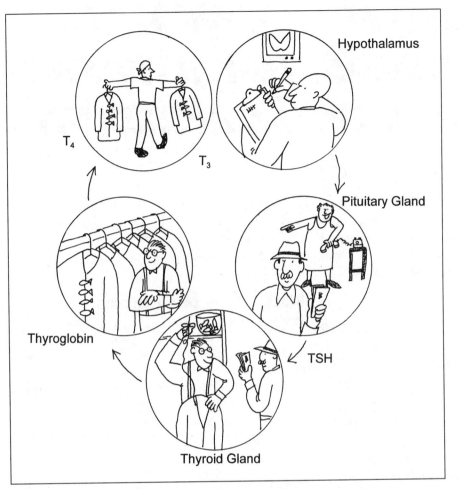

■ Fig. 25-3 ■
Action of thyroid
stimulating hormone.

Liothyronine (Cytomel and Cytomine) has a short half-life and hence is used diagnostically in the T_3 suppression test.

Liotrix (Euthyroid, Thyrolar) is a combination of T_4 and T_3, and is standardized to yield a T_4 to T_3 ratio of 4 to 1.

Treatment of Myxedema Coma

If hypothyroidism goes untreated, myxedema coma results. It is characterized by hypothermia (75°F, 24°C), hypoglycemia, bradycardia, and hypotension. Alveolar hypotension may lead to hypoxia, followed by lethargy, coma, and death. Treatment includes:

- Administration of a loading dose of levothyroxine (300–400 μg IV)
- Administration of a daily dose of levothyroxine (50 μg)
- Maintenance of respiration with mechanical ventilation and assisted oxygen administration
- Evaluation of adrenocortical insufficiency and the administration of corticosteroids
- Hypertonic saline and glucose therapy to alleviate hyponatremia and hypoglycemia

In addition, any other supportive therapy should be instituted as indicated.

CHAPTER 26

Vitamin D, Calcium Homeostasis, Parathyroid Hormone, and Calcitonin

Four **parathyroid glands,** situated on the lateral lobes of the thyroid, secrete **parathyroid hormone** in response to low serum calcium levels. Parathyroid hormone then increases the serum calcium levels through the functioning of several mechanisms:

- It stimulates bone resorption.
- It increases the intestinal absorption of calcium.
- It increases the resorption of calcium by the renal tubules.
- It acts on the kidney to decrease the tubular resorption of phosphate.

A reciprocal relationship exists between the level of calcium and phosphorus, as shown in ■ **Table 26-1** ■ and ■ **Fig. 26-1** ■

Calcitonin is also involved in calcium homeostasis; it inhibits bone resorption and prevents excess increases in the serum calcium concentration through its monitoring of parathyroid hormone's actions. See ■ **Fig. 26-1** ■

Function of Calcium Ions

Calcium functions at both extracellular and cellular sites. Its **extracellular functions** consist of:

- Maintenance of normal ion products for mineralization
- Cofactor for prothrombin and factors VII, IX, and X
- Maintenance of plasma membrane stability and permeability

Its **cellular functions** comprise:

- Skeletal and cardiac muscle contraction
- Cellular secretion (exocrine, endocrine, and neurotransmitters)
- Neural excitation and light transmission

- Regulation of membrane ion transport
- Enzyme regulation (gluconeogenesis and glycogenolysis)
- Cell growth and division

Biosynthesis of Calcitonin

The primary stimulus for calcitonin synthesis and secretion is an increase in the serum concentration of **ionized calcium.** Calcitonin secretion has been found to be uninfluenced by parathyroid hormone, 25-hydroxyvitamin D, thyroid-stimulating hormone, pregnancy, or lactation.

Vitamin D

Vitamins D_3 and D_2 are produced by ultraviolet irradiation of animal skin and plants, respectively. The precursor of vitamin D_3 in skin is 7-dehyrocholesterol, or **provitamin D.**

Parathyroid Hormone Disorders

Hypoparathyroidism

Hypocalcemic tetany is treated with the IV administration of **calcium gluconate** or **calcium chloride** (5–10 ml of 10% solution). The effects of these agents are rapid but transient. ■ **Fig. 26-2** ■ Because

■ **Table 26-1** ■ The Effects of Parathyroid Hormone on Serum Levels of Calcium and Phosphate

Disorder	Serum Calcium	Serum Phosphate
Hyperparathyroidism	Elevated	Low
Hypoparathyroidism	Low	Elevated

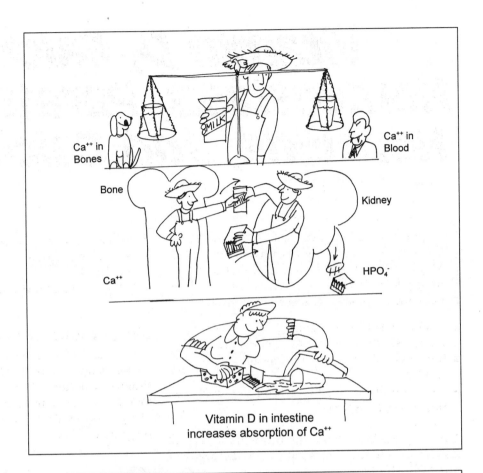

■ Fig. 26-1 ■

Actions of parathyroid hormone.

■ Fig. 26-2 ■

Drugs altering the level of calcium.

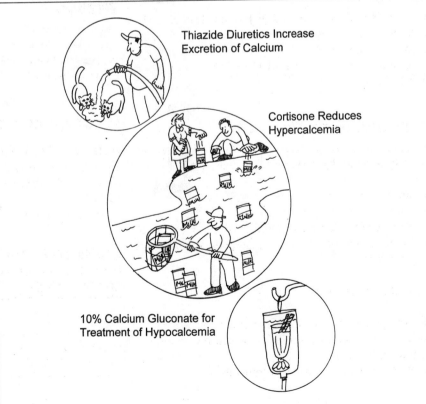

calcium chloride is a highly irritating substance, it should not be administered intramuscularly. Parathyroid hormone (100–300 units) is injected subcutaneously after the initial administration of calcium salt, but its effect is transient and lasts only 3–4 weeks. Hypoparathyroidism is also treated with vitamin D (1–2 mg, or 50,000–100,000 units per day). ■ **Fig. 26-3** ■

Hyperparathyroidism

Hyperparathyroidism is treated surgically. Prior to surgery, patients may be treated with corticosteroids to antagonize the vitamin D–induced intestinal absorption of calcium and also increase calcium excretion by the kidney. See ■ **Fig. 26-2** ■

Osteoporosis

Osteoporosis, which is predominantly seen in women, has been linked to a lack of estrogen and decreased intestinal absorption of calcium. The administration of corticosteroids causes an excess resorption of bone and excretion of calcium in the urine. See ■ **Fig. 26-2** ■ Other drugs that adversely affect bone metabolism are **phenytoin, barbiturates, thyroxine, heparin,** and certain **loop diuretics.** Calcium supplements in combination with estrogen therapy have been used to prevent and treat postmenopausal osteoporosis. In addition, **alendronate sodium** (fosamax), which decreases the faster rate of bone loss, may be used in women after menopause.

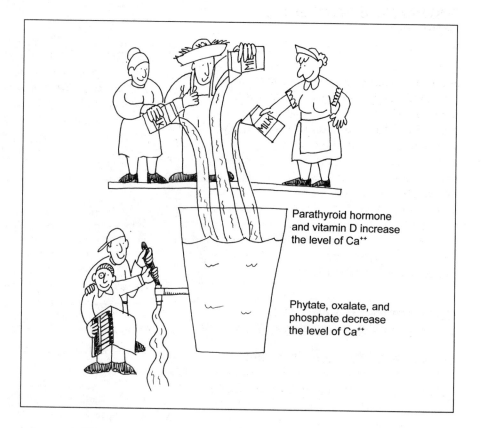

Parathyroid hormone and vitamin D increase the level of Ca⁺⁺

Phytate, oxalate, and phosphate decrease the level of Ca⁺⁺

■ **Fig. 26-3** ■
Substances altering the level of calcium.

CHAPTER 27

Hypothalamic and Pituitary Hormones

Hypothalamic peptides released into the hypothalamic-hypophyseal portal circulation provide the means by which the CNS communicates with the anterior pituitary and the peripheral endocrine organs.

Gonadotropin-Releasing Hormone

The pituitary hormones responsible for regulating gonadal functions are **luteinizing hormone** (LH) and **follicle-stimulating hormone** (FSH). In **males,** LH stimulates the Leydig's cells to synthesize **testosterone;** FSH stimulates the Sertoli's cells to synthesize **inhibin** and **androgen-binding protein** and, in conjunction with high intratesticular concentrations of testosterone, initiates and maintains **spermatogenesis. In females,** LH stimulates **androgen synthesis,** and FSH increases estrogen and inhibin synthesis in the granulosa cells. Both LH and FSH are released from the gonadotroph cells of the anterior pituitary in response to the hypothalamic hormone gonadotropin-releasing hormone (GnRH; also known as **LH-releasing hormone**).

Gonadotropin-Releasing Hormone Replacement Therapy

Induction of Puberty in Males

GnRH is used to induce puberty in males with **idiopathic hypogonadotropic hypogonadism** (IHH). Gonadotropin-releasing hormone (15–150 ng/kg per hour) is administered by an infusion pump that delivers GnRH as a bolus, but in a pulsatile fashion. This induces the secretion of LH and FSH, the level of testosterone rises, the size of the testes increases, and spermatogenesis commences.

Induction of Ovulation in Females

Gonadotropin-releasing hormone is used in females to treat **hypothalamic amenorrhea.** A deficit in the synthesis of GnRH has been implicated as the source of menstrual disturbances, hypoprolactinemia, anorexia nervosa, stress- and weight-loss-associated amenorrhea, athletes' amenorrhea, some forms of the polycystic ovarian disease syndrome, and infertility associated with hypothalamic tumors.

Growth Hormone-Releasing Hormone

Growth hormone is secreted in a pulsatile fashion during sleep by the somatotrophs of the anterior pituitary gland. Two hypothalamic peptides, **growth hormone-releasing hormone** (GHRH) and **somatostatin** (somatotropin release-inhibiting hormone), are the principal stimulatory and inhibitory factors of GHRH, respectively. **Growth hormone deficiency** in children causes short stature, which will respond to GHRH replacement therapy.

Oxytocin

The direct stimulatory effect of oxytocin is prominent in the gravid uterus during the late stage of pregnancy. Its action is augmented by estrogen and inhibited by progesterone. Oxytocin's effect is specific for uterine muscle; little effect is observed on intestinal muscle or coronary arteries. Oxytocin (Pitocin, Syntocinon, and Uteracon) is used for the following purposes:

- To **induce term labor,** although it may be contraindicated during the first and second stages of labor
- To **control postpartum hemorrhage**
- To **prevent postpartum uterine atony**
- To **expel the placenta**
- To **prevent postpartum breast engorgement** in some women by stimulating milk letdown. The suckling stimulus initiates a neurogenic reflex that is transmitted through the spinal cord, midbrain, and hypothalamus, where it mediates the release of oxytocin and finally lactation. Pain, stress, and adrenergic agonists are known to retard milk letdown. ■ **Fig. 27-1** ■

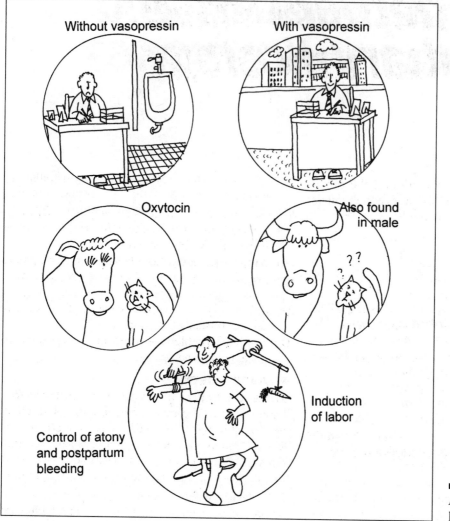

Without vasopressin

With vasopressin

Oxytocin

Also found in male

Control of atony and postpartum bleeding

Induction of labor

■ **Fig. 27-1** ■
Actions of pituitary hormones.

Vasopressin

The second hormone that originates from the posterior pituitary gland is **antidiuretic hormone,** or **vasopressin.**

Vasopressin Deficiency

The loss of the neurosecretory neurons that make up the neurohypophysis eliminates the secretion of vasopressin, and this produces **diabetes insipidus.** See ■ **Fig. 27-1** ■ Agents that cause the syndrome of inappropriate antidiuretic secretion consist of: carbamazepine, chlorpropamide, clofibrate, cyclophosphamide, haloperidol, monoamine oxidase inhibitors, nicotine, oxytocin, phenothiazine derivatives, thiazide diuretics, tricyclic antidepressants, vasopressin, and vincristine.

Vasopressin Preparations

Vasopressin (Pitressin) may be administered either subcutaneously or intramuscularly. It has a duration of action of 2–8 hours. Vasopressin tannate (Pitressin Tannate) is a suspension and should be injected intramuscularly only. It has a duration action of 2–3 days. **Desmopressin acetate** is used topically. **Lypressin** (Diapid) is administered as an intranasal spray. All of these agents may be used in the treatment of central diabetes insipidus (vasopressin sensitive).

CHAPTER 28

Reproductive Pharmacology

In the absence of pituitary gonadotropins, the gonads fail to develop properly, and removal of the pituitary gland causes reproductive failure.

Estrogens

Estrogens are synthesized mainly in the ovaries, the placenta, and the adrenal glands. A minute amount of estradiol is synthesized in the testes. Estrogens are synthesized according to the following scheme.

Cholesterol → pregnenolone → progesterone → androstenedione → estradiol 17 beta → estrone → estriol

Physiologic Actions

Estrogen dramatically influences the growth and development of the **female reproductive organs.**

Therapeutic Uses of Estrogen Preparations

The estrogen preparations are basically divided into three groups: natural steroids, semisynthetic steroids, and nonsteroidal chemical compounds possessing estrogenic activities. **Transdermal estrogen** (Estraderm) equals the efficacy of the oral preparation.

Estrogens are used extensively in the treatment of endocrine and nonendocrine diseases, a few of which are cited below:

Menopause — as a replacement therapy
Atrophic vaginitis — to thicken epithelial cells and to cause mucosal cells to proliferate
Hypopituitarism — to correct vaginal mucosal atrophy, maintain breast development, and minimize calcium loss from bone
Cancer — used in postmenopausal mammary carcinoma
Primary hypogonadism — to correct ovarian failure
Osteoporosis — in the treatment of osteoporosis, either by itself or with hypercalcemic steroid

Primary amenorrhea — to cause endometrium to proliferate
Uterine bleeding — to reverse estrogen deficiency (oral contraceptives containing 80–100 µg of estrogen are recommended)
Postpartum lactation — to relieve postpartum painful breast engorgement and prevent postpartum lactation (bromocriptine is also effective)
Control of height — to cause closure of the epiphyses in unusually tall young girls
Dermatologic problems — used in the treatment of acne, with some success

Adverse Effects

Low-dose estrogens are safe only when taken for a limited period. The most often reported side effects are breakthrough bleeding, breast tenderness, and very infrequent GI upsets. When estrogens are used in large doses or injudiciously, they may cause thromboembolic disorders, hypertension in susceptible individuals, and cholestasis.

Estrogens are contraindicated in patients with estrogen-dependent neoplasms such as carcinoma of the breast or endometrium. **Vaginal adenocarcinoma** has been reported in young women whose mothers were treated with **diethylstilbestrol** in an effort to prevent miscarriage.

Antiestrogens

Clomiphene (Clomid) and **tamoxifen** (Nolvadex) modify the actions of estrogens. They accomplish this by binding to the cytoplasmic estrogen receptors that are then translocated to the nucleus. Antiestrogens are able to arrest the growth of estrogen-dependent malignant mammary cells. Clomiphene has been used in certain cases of disseminated breast cancer.

Progesterone and Progestins

Progesterone is synthesized by the ovaries, the adrenal glands, and the placenta. In a nonpregnant woman, it is produced by the **corpus luteum** during the latter part of the menstrual cycle under the influence of luteinizing and luteotropic hormones. In a pregnant woman, it is produced initially by the corpus luteum under the influence of chorionic gonadotropins and is synthesized by the **placenta** after failure of the corpus luteum.

Progesterone is not only an important **progestin** but also an important precursor for androgen. It is synthesized according to the following scheme:

$$Acetate \rightarrow cholesterol \rightarrow pregnenolone \rightarrow progesterone \rightarrow testosterone \rightarrow estradiol$$

Therapeutic Uses

Progestins are used as **antifertility agents** and in the treatment of **dysfunctional uterine bleeding,** which may occur as a result of insufficient estrogen or because of continued estrogen secretion in the absence of progesterone.

Amenorrhea - Progestins such as **medroxyprogesterone** are useful in the diagnosis and treatment of amenorrhea.

Dysmenorrhea - Because **prostaglandin F_{2a}** is capable of inducing contraction in the uterus, agents that are able to block the synthesis of prostaglandin, such as **aspirin** or aspirin-like substances, have been shown to be effective in easing dysmenorrhea. For sexually active women, oral contraceptives have been found to be effective in relieving dysmenorrhea.

Endometriosis - Endometriosis, which was formerly treated by surgical removal of the ovaries and uterus, is now treated with the continuous administration of progestin or with progestin combined with estrogen. In addition, progestin may be useful in the management of **endometrial carcinoma.**

Suppression of Postpartum Lactation - Estrogen, progesterone, and bromocriptine (a dopamine receptor agonist) are all effective in suppressing postpartum lactation.

Antifertility Agents

Mechanism of Action

The antifertility agents suppress ovulation by:

- Inhibiting the release of hypophyseal ovulation-regulating gonadotropin

- Producing thick mucus from the cervical glands and hence impeding the penetration of sperm cells into the uterus
- Impeding the transfer of the ovum from the oviduct to the uterus
- Preventing implantation of the fertilized ovum should fertilization take place

Side Effects

Breast Cancer - There is no evidence for either an increase or decrease in the risk of breast cancer among users of oral contraceptives.

Cervical Cancer - There is an increased incidence of dysplasia of the cervix, epidermoid carcinoma, and adenocarcinoma among users of oral contraceptives as compared with matched control groups.

Endometrial Cancer - Oral contraceptives seem to protect against endometrial cancer.

Ovarian Cancer - The use of oral contraceptives reduces the risk of ovarian cancer.

Liver Adenoma and Cancer - The development of a benign hepatocellular adenoma is a rare occurrence among long-term users of oral contraceptives.

Pituitary Adenoma - The incidence of pituitary adenoma among users of oral contraceptives is not higher than that seen among matched controls.

Reproductive Effects - The rate of return of fertility after the discontinued use of contraceptives is lower for users of oral contraceptives than that for women who have used barrier methods for 2–3 years.

Androgens

Testosterone, the male sex hormone, is responsible for the development and maintenance of the **male sex organs** (the penis, prostate gland, seminal vessicle, and vas deferens) and **secondary sex characteristics.**

Therapeutic Uses

Testosterone and its derivatives are used in the treatment of hypogonadism (eunuchoidism), hypopituitarism, accelerated growth, aging in men, osteoporosis, anemia, endometriosis, promotion of anabolism, suppression of lactation, and breast carcinoma.

Hormonal therapy with testosterone should be reserved primarily for patients with **hypogonadal disorders.**

Side Effects

One of the side effects of testosterone compounds is **masculinization in women** (such as hirsutism, acne, depression of menses, and clitoral enlargement) and of their female offspring. Therefore, androgens are contraindicated in pregnant women. **Prostatic hypertrophy** may occur in males, which leads to urinary retention. Therefore, androgens are contraindicated in men with **prostatic carcinoma.**

Antiandrogens

Cyproterone inhibits the action of androgens, and **gossypol** prevents spermatogenesis without altering the other endocrine functions of the testis.

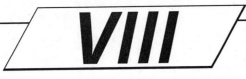

VIII

Gastrointestinal and Pulmonary Pharmacology

CHAPTER 29

Gastrointestinal Pharmacology

Acid Pepsin Disease

The medical treatment of esophageal, gastric, and duodenal ulcers includes relieving the symptoms, accelerating healing, preventing complications, and preventing recurrence. **Drug treatment** includes the use of antacids, anticholinergic drugs, histamine H_2-receptor antagonists, inhibitors of H^+K^+ ATPase, and antibiotics to eradicate *Helicobacter pylori*.

Drug Therapy

Antacids

Because acid-pepsin disease rarely occurs in the absence of gastric acid and pepsin, antacids are highly effective in its overall management. Antacids consist of a mixture of magnesium, aluminum, and calcium compounds. Their efficacy is based on their inherent ability to **react with and neutralize gastric acid. Sodium bicarbonate,** which may leave the stomach rapidly, can cause alkalosis and sodium retention. **Calcium salts** may produce hypercalcemia, which can be detrimental in patients with impaired renal function. **Aluminum salts** may decrease the absorption of tetracyclines and anticholinergic drugs.

Anticholinergic Drugs

Vagal impulses elicit the release of acetylcholine in the parietal cells and in the gastric mucosal cells containing **gastrin,** a peptide hormone. Both the directly released acetylcholine and the indirectly released gastrin then stimulate the parietal cells to secrete hydrogen ions into the gastric lumen.

The most useful anticholinergic drugs are **propantheline** (Pro-Banthine), **pirenzepine,** and **telenzepine,** which antagonize muscarinic cholinergic receptors. All three agents depress gastric motility and secretion. The production of pepsin is also reduced. Propantheline may be used as adjunctive therapy with antacids but not as a sole agent. The side effects and contraindications of propantheline use are identical to those of atropine (prostatic hypertrophy, urinary retention, glaucoma, and cardiac arrhythmias).

The **timing** of medication is critical in ulcer therapy. Anticholinergic drugs should be given about 30 minutes before meals and antacids about 1 hour after meals. A double dose of an antacid is often taken just before bedtime.

Histamine H_2-Receptor Antagonists

There are two types of histamine receptors: **H_1 receptors,** which are blocked by agents such as diphenhydramine and other antiallergic compounds, and **H_2 receptors,** which are blocked by cimetidine (Tagamet), ranitidine (Zantac), famotidine (Pepcid), and nizatidine (Axid). Cimetidine has no effect on most H_1-receptor-mediated effects, such as bronchoconstriction. ■ **Fig. 29-1** ■

The clinical use of H_2-receptor antagonists stems from their capacity to inhibit gastric acid secretion, especially in patients with peptic ulceration. **Cimetidine,** which is far more efficacious than anticholinergic drugs, is used in the treatment of duodenal ulcers and gastrinoma, and in patients suffering from gastroesophageal reflux. It is absorbed orally, has a plasma half-life of 2 hours, and is excreted mainly unchanged by the kidney. The doses of cimetidine must be reduced in the presence of impaired renal function. The few and infrequent **adverse effects** of cimetidine use include gynecomastia (may bind to androgen receptor sites), galactorrhea (especially in patients with gastrinoma), granulocytopenia, agranulocytosis (very rare), mental confusion (especially in the elderly), restlessness, seizures, and reduced sperm count. **Ranitidine** is more effective than cimetidine and allegedly has fewer side effects.

Inhibitors of H^+K^+ ATPase

The **proton pump** (H^+K^+ ATPase) of the apical membrane of the parietal cells is the ultimate mechanism that governs acid secretion. Among a family of benzimidazole derivatives, **omeprazole** (Losec)

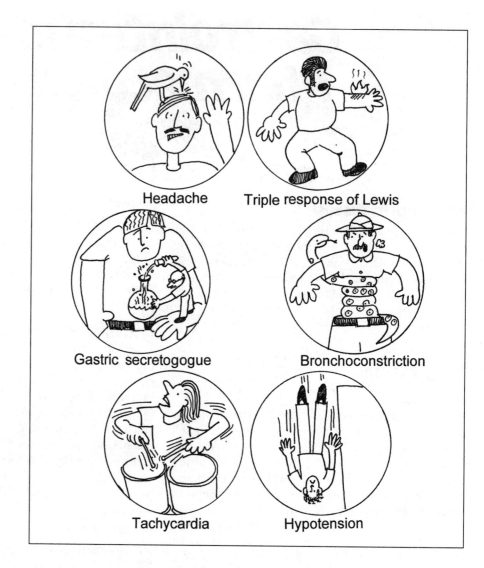

■ Fig. 29-1 ■
Actions of histamine.

promotes the healing of ulcers in the stomach, duodenum, and esophagus, and is of special value in patients who do not respond to H_2-receptor antagonists.

Eradication of *Helicobacter Pylori*

Helicobacter pylori is a gram-negative rod that colonizes the mucus on the luminal surface of the gastric epithelium. *H. pylori* infection causes an inflammatory gastritis and is a putative contributor to peptic ulcer disease, gastric lymphoma, and adenocarcinoma. Both **amoxicillin** and **clarithromycin** are effective in some patients. Because of resistance developed by *H. pylori,* multiple drugs are needed.

Nausea and Vomiting Antiemetic Agents

Agents That Block Dopamine Receptors

The nausea and vomiting associated with circulating physical agents (radiation therapy and virus particles) and chemical agents (toxins and cancer chemotherapeutic agents) are treated with phenothiazine derivatives such as chlorpromazine, perphenazine, prochlorperazine, promethazine, triethylperazine, and triflupromazine. These agents block the dopamine receptors in the **area postrema. ■ Fig. 29-2 ■**

Agents That Block Serotonin Receptors

A new class of antiemetic agents, the serotonin receptor antagonists, has been identified. These agents could

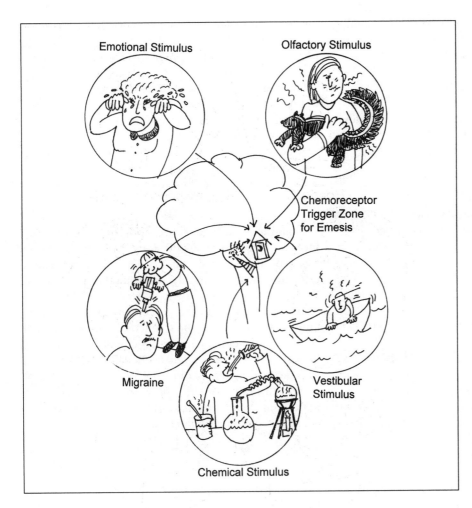

Emotional Stimulus

Olfactory Stimulus

Chemoreceptor
Trigger Zone
for Emesis

Migraine

Vestibular
Stimulus

Chemical Stimulus

■ Fig. 29-2 ■
Activation of the chemo-receptor trigger zone for emesis by various stimuli.

be clinically useful in a wide range of areas. Selective antagonists of the serotonin (5-hydroxytryptamine) type 3 (5-HT$_3$) receptor such as **batanopride, granisetron, ondansetron,** or **zacopride** have proved in early clinical trials to be potent antiemetic agents in patients undergoing cytotoxic chemotherapy. Their efficacy has been shown to be comparable or superior to that of conventional phenothiazine antiemetics. The toxic effects observed so far with these agents have been modest.

Laxatives and Cathartics

Constipation may be defined as the passage of excessively dry stools, infrequent stools, or stools of insufficient size. Constipation is a symptom, not a disease.

Irritants

Irritant agents used in the treatment of constipation include cascara sagrada, castor oil, senna, rhubarb, phenolphthalein, and acetphenolisatin.

Phenolphthalein is thought to exert its effect by inhibiting the movement of water and sodium from the colon into the blood and by stimulating mucus secretion. **Castor oil** is hydrolyzed to **ricinoleic acid,** the active cathartic. It has an onset of action of 2–6 hours.

Bulk Saline Laxatives

Bulk saline laxatives fall into two categories: **inorganic salts** (magnesium sulfate, magnesium citrate, milk of magnesia, sodium sulfate, and sodium phosphate) and **organic hydrophilic colloids** (methylcellulose, carboxymethylcellulose [Metamucil], plantage seed, agar, psyllium, bran, and fruits). They exert their effects by absorbing and retaining water, increasing bulk, stimulating colonic peristaltic movements, and lubricating and hydrating the desiccated fecal materials.

Lubricants

The lubricants consist of mineral oil and dioctyl sodium sulfosuccinate (docusate). They are used in the pharmaceutical industry as an emulsifying and dispersing substance. Both agents are taken orally. These agents, which do not influence peristalsis, soften desiccated stools or delay the desiccation of fecal materials.

Other Uses of Laxatives

Poisoning - Laxatives are used to hasten the elimination and reduce the absorption of a poison that has been taken.

Antihelminthics - Laxatives are used before and after treatment with antihelminthic drugs.

Radiology - Laxatives are used to clean the GI tract before radiographic techniques are performed.

Diarrhea

The treatment of diarrhea consists of the following:

- Fluid replenishment is accomplished through the consumption of liquids and salty food.
- Antiinflammatory agents such as prednisone may be effective for treating diarrhea associated with bowel disease.
- Hypolipoproteinemic substances such as cholestyramine, which binds bile acid in the intestine, have

been used in controlling the diarrhea associated with bile acid malabsorption.

- Neuroleptics such as phenothiazine derivatives inhibit the intestinal secretion caused by cholera toxin and *Escherichia coli* enterotoxins.
- Bismuth subsalicylate prevents and diminishes infection with enterotoxin-producing *E. coli*.
- Local anesthetic ointments may be helpful when used for a short time in the symptomatic treatment of perianal discomfort.
- Opioids may have a place in treatment (see Chap. 10).

The antidiarrheal agents are **codeine, diphenoxylate** and **atropine** (Lomotil), and loperamide. Because it causes less addiction than codeine, **loperamide** is now the most commonly used antidiarrheal agent. These agents achieve their effects by reducing the propulsive activity of the gut, enhancing the contact time between the intestinal mucosal and the luminal contents, and enhancing active chloride absorption, hence opposing the secretory effects of toxin. Opioid antidiarrheal agents should not be used in cases of severe ulcerative colitis threatened by impending toxic megacolon or in patients with shigellosis because they prolong duration of the disease.

CHAPTER 30

Pulmonary Pharmacology

Drugs Used in the Treatment of Asthma

Cyclic Adenosine Monophosphate and Bronchial Asthma

Cyclic adenosine monophosphate (cAMP) prevents bronchial smooth muscle contraction, promotes bronchial smooth muscle relaxation, and inhibits the release of mediators. The metabolism of cAMP takes place according to the following scheme:

$$\text{Adenosine triphosphate} \xrightarrow{\text{Adenylate cyclase}} \text{cAMP} \xrightarrow{\text{Phosphodiesterase}} 5' \text{ AMP}$$

Agents that stimulate the activity of adenylate cyclase (beta$_2$ agonists), inhibit the activity of phosphodiesterase (aminophylline), or enhance the effects of beta$_2$ agonists on their receptor sites (corticosteroids) are extremely useful **antiasthmatic agents.** Conversely, substances that block the beta-adrenergic receptor sites (propranolol) or that stimulate either the cholinergic receptor sites (cholinomimetic agents) or the alpha-adrenergic receptor site (prostaglandin F$_{2a}$) cause **bronchoconstriction.** Furthermore, the muscarinic cholinergic receptor agonists (ipratropium bromide) are potential **bronchodilators.** ■ Fig. 30-1 ■

Methylxanthine Drugs

The methylxanthines consist of **aminophylline, dyphylline, enprofylline,** and **pentoxifylline.** Aminophylline (theophylline, ethylendiamine) is the most widely used of the soluble theophyllines. Its main therapeutic effect is bronchodilation. In addition, it causes CNS stimulation, cardiac acceleration, diuresis, and gastric secretion. Aminophylline is available in an oral, rectal (pediatric), or IV solution, which is used in the treatment of status asthmaticus. Although aminophylline is a less effective bronchodilator than beta-adrenergic agonists, it is particularly useful in preventing nocturnal asthma.

Bronchodilators

Bronchodilators are sympathomimetic agents that stimulate beta-receptor sites. The most effective of these are beta-adrenergic receptor agonists, which activate adenylate cyclase, thus increasing the concentration of cAMP, which inhibits the hydrolysis of phosphoinositide. Theophylline increases the concentration of cAMP by inhibiting the activity of phosphodiesterase.

Epinephrine

Epinephrine may be used subcutaneously in the treatment of status asthmaticus. It has a rapid onset of action of 3–5 minutes and a short duration of action of 15–20 minutes.

Selective Beta$_2$ Stimulants

The selective beta$_2$-adrenergic stimulants cause bronchodilation without cardiac acceleration. **Metaproterenol** and **terbutaline** are available in tablet form, and terbutaline is also available for subcutaneous injection. Metaproterenol and **albuterol** are available in metered-dose inhalers. See ■ Fig. 30-1 ■

Inhaled selective beta$_2$-adrenergic receptor agonists (**albuterol, terbutaline, fenoterol,** and **bitolterol**) have a rapid onset of action and are effective for 3–6 hours. **Formoterol** and **salmeterol** are longer-acting agents (12 hours) and may prove useful in treating nocturnal symptoms.

The **side effects** of beta-adrenergic receptor agonists are tremor, tachycardias, and palpitations.

Anticholinergic Bronchodilators

Ipratropium bromide (Atrovent) is a congener of atropine. It works as a bronchodilator by inhibiting the cholinergic activation of airway smooth muscle. Less potent than adrenergic agonists, it is useful in patients with chronic bronchitis and emphysema. See ■ Fig. 30-1 ■

Cromolyn Sodium and Nedocromil Sodium

Cromolyn sodium is given by inhalation as an aerosol powder four times a day only as a prophylactic medication. Since it is not a bronchodilator, it is not used in the management of status asthmaticus. Because it

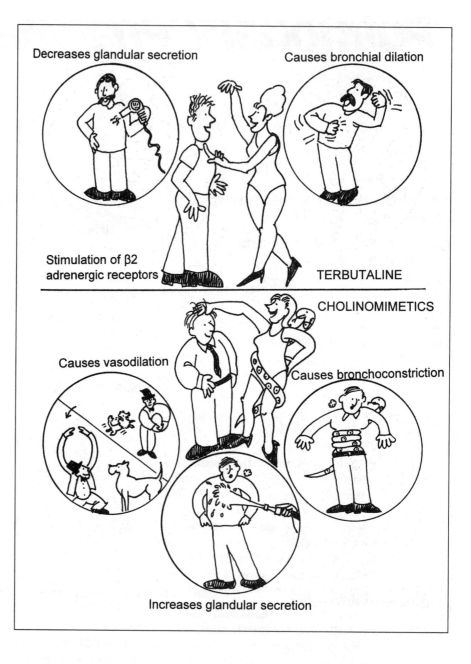

Decreases glandular secretion

Causes bronchial dilation

Stimulation of β2 adrenergic receptors

TERBUTALINE

CHOLINOMIMETICS

Causes vasodilation

Causes bronchoconstriction

Increases glandular secretion

■ Fig. 30-1 ■
Drugs indicated or contra-indicated in asthma.

can inhibit the immediate response to allergens or exercise, it is thought that it suppresses the release of the mediators from mast cells. Cromolyn also prevents the late response and the subsequent hypersecretion, and this suggests it acts on other inflammatory cells such as macrophages or eosinophils. Cromolyn is not effective in all patients. It is the preferred antiinflammatory agent for use in children. The drug is well tolerated and, with the exception of causing minor throat irritation, has no side effects. **Nedocromil sodium** (Tilade) has biologic

and chemical properties similar to those of cromolyn sodium. **■ Fig. 30-2 ■**

Corticosteroids

Prednisone is available in oral form, and **beclomethasone** may be used as an aerosol, especially in children. The corticosteroids may exert their effects through multiple mechanisms, including:

■ Relaxing bronchospasm
■ Decreasing mucus secretion
■ Potentiating beta-adrenergic receptors

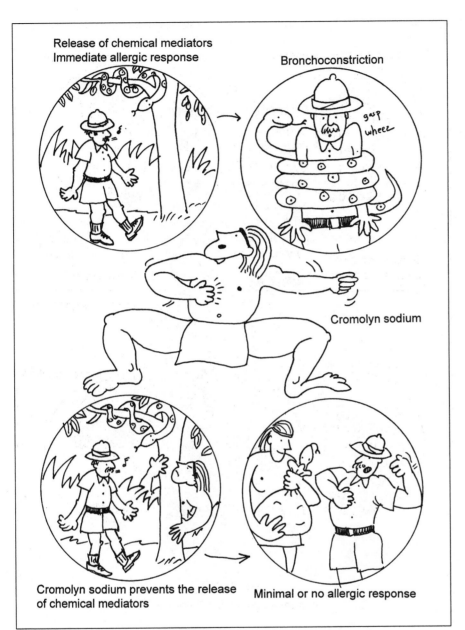

Release of chemical mediators
Immediate allergic response

Bronchoconstriction

Cromolyn sodium

Cromolyn sodium prevents the release
of chemical mediators

Minimal or no allergic response

■ **Fig. 30-2** ■
Beneficial effects of
cromolyn sodium.

- Stabilizing lysosomes
- Possessing antiinflammatory properties
- Inhibiting antibody formation
- Antagonizing histamine actions

Corticosteroids do not inhibit the release of mediators from mast cells or block the early response to allergens, but they do block the late response and the subsequent bronchial hyperresponsiveness.

Steroids such as **beclomethasone dipropionate, budesonide, trimcinolone acetonide,** and **flu-nisolide** are active when given topically and can control asthma without causing systemic effects or adrenal suppression. However, orally administered steroids, such as **prednisone, prednisolone,** or **methylprednisolone** are still needed by some patients.

The **side effects** of high-dose inhalational steroids include oropharyngeal candidiasis and dysphonia. The orally administered steroids may produce osteoporosis, weight gain, hypertension, diabetes, myopathy, psychiatric disturbances, skin fragility, or cataracts.

Antitussive Medications

The antitussive medications fall into two categories: **narcotic** (e.g., codeine) and **nonnarcotic** (e.g., dextromethorphan and levopropoxyphene).

Codeine

Most narcotics (such as **morphine, codeine, dihydrocodeinone, methadone,** and **levorphanol**) have antitussive properties. Codeine is used primarily because its addictive liability is low, and it is effective orally. The antitussive doses of narcotics are lower than the doses used for analgesic purposes.

Dextromethorphan

Dextromethorphan (Romilar), like codeine, exerts its antitussive action by elevating the cough threshold in the medulla. Unlike codeine, dextromethorphan has no respiratory depressant, analgesic, or addictive properties. Furthermore, it does not cause drowsiness, narcosis, or GI irritation.

Mucolytic Agents

Actylcysteine (Mucomyst) is the most widely used mucolytic drug.

Mucokinetic Agents

Ammonium chloride, ammonium carbonate, potassium citrate, potassium iodide, ipecac, creosotes, guaicols, and volatile oils (oils of anise, eucalyptus, lemon, pine, and turpentine) are all expectorants.

IX

Pharmacology of Signal Transduction and the Second-Messenger System

CHAPTER 31

Autacoids

Histamine and Antihistamines

In the peripheral system, histamine causes:

- Capillary dilation and increased permeability
- Bronchoconstriction and contraction of GI muscles
- Stimulation of chromaffin cells releasing catecholamines
- Vasodilation, tachycardia, and headache
- Stimulation of exocrine secretion causing hypersecretion of mucus in the lungs
- Stimulation of gastric secretion See ■ **Fig. 29-1** ■

Agents Interacting with Various Histamine Receptor Subtypes

The diversified actions of histamine are brought forth through their interaction with different types of receptors.

Histamine₁ Receptors

Histamine$_1$ (H$_1$) receptors mediate such actions as bronchoconstriction and the contraction of smooth muscles in the GI tract. These effects are blocked by classic antihistaminics such as diphenhydramine hydrochloride (Benadryl).

Terfenadine, astemizole, loratadine, and **cetirizine** are **second-generation** antihistaminic agents that are relatively **nonsedating.** Other H$_1$-receptor antagonists are **azelastine, ebastine,** and **levocabastine.**

Histamine₂ Receptors

Stimulation of the H$_2$ receptors elicits a variety of responses, the most widely studied of which is **gastric acid secretion** from the parietal cells of the gastric glands. However, many other effects mediated by H$_2$ receptors are manifested in peripheral tissues. These include the positive chronotropic action in the auricular muscle, the inotropic action in the ventricular muscle, and the lipolytic effect in fat cells. Examples of the various H$_2$-receptor blocking agents are:

Imidazole derivatives: Cimetidine and etintidine
Furan derivatives: Ranitidine and nizatidine

Guanidinothiazole derivatives: Famotidine
Piperidinomethylphenoxy derivatives: Roxatidine acetate and roxatidine

Histamine₃ Receptors

H$_3$ receptors suppress **gastric acid secretion,** and this is evoked by cholinergic stimuli. H$_3$ receptors exist outside the parietal cells and seem to be located on cholinergic and nonadrenergic neurons of the myenteric plexus, where they inhibit the release of neurotransmitters. The agonist and antagonist for H$_3$ receptors are **alpha-methylhistamine** and **thioperamide,** respectively.

Adenosine

As an autacoid, adenosine:

- Possesses negative chronotropic and inotropic effects
- Is a vasodilator in almost all vascular beds
- Inhibits neurotransmitter release in the CNS
- Causes sedation
- Displays anticonvulsant activity
- Regulates renin release
- Inhibits platelet aggregation
- Modulates lymphocyte function
- Induces bronchospasm
- Inhibits lipolysis

Receptors for adenosine, referred to as **purinergic receptors** (P$_1$), should be distinguished from the P$_2$ receptors that mediate the actions of adenosine triphosphate in the GI tract and vascular endothelium. The adenosine receptors are further classified as P$_1$A$_2$, which activate adenyl cyclase, and P$_1$A$_1$, which inhibit adenyl cyclase.

Serotonin

Serotonin Receptors and Their Subtypes

Ligand-binding studies and molecular biologic examination of membrane preparations have revealed that there are at least fourteen types of serotonin receptors, including $5\text{-}HT_{1A}$, $5\text{-}HT_{1B}$, $5\text{-}HT_{1C}$, $5\text{-}HT_{1D}$, $5\text{-}HT_{1E}$, $5\text{-}HT_{1F}$, $5\text{-}HT_{2A}$ (D receptor), $5\text{-}HT_{2B}$, $5\text{-}HT_{2C}$, $5\text{-}H_{T3}$ (M receptor), $5\text{-}HT_4$, $5\text{-}HT_{5B}$, $5\text{-}HT_6$, and $5\text{-}HT_7$ receptor subtypes.

Actions of Serotonin

Serotonin possesses many actions. It:

- Is involved in the neural network that regulates intestinal motility
- Is released by a carcinoid
- Is released by platelets (also adenosine diphosphate) during aggregation
- Causes vasoconstriction by stimulating $5HT_2$ receptors, and this effect is blocked by **ketanserine**
- Causes vasodilation by stimulating $5HT_1$ receptors
- Causes positive inotropic and chronotropic effects by interacting with both $5HT_1$ and $5HT_3$ receptors
- Increases the motility of the stomach as well as small and large intestines
- Causes uterine contractions
- Causes bronchial contractions

Serotonin Receptor Antagonists

Ketanserine, a $5\text{-}HT_2$ and alpha$_1$-adrenergic receptor antagonist, lowers blood pressure.

Methysergide, a $5\text{-}HT_{1C}$ antagonist, has been used for the prophylactic treatment of migraine and other vascular headache, including **Horton's syndrome.** Calcium entry blockers such as **flunarizine** have been shown to be effective in treating migraine.

Cyprohepadine, a serotonin and histamine$_1$ receptor- and muscarinic cholinergic receptor-blocking agent, has been used in the treatment of the **postgastrectomy dumping syndrome** and the intestinal hypermotility seen with carcinoid.

Sumatriptan, an agonist of the $5\text{-}HT_{1D}$-like receptor, is highly effective in the treatment of migraine.

Ondansetron, granisetron, tropisetron, and **batanopride** are antagonists of the $5HT_3$ receptor and are considered effective in controlling cancer chemotherapy–induced emesis.

Clozapine, an effective antipsychotic agent with little or no extrapyramidal side effects, has a high affinity for $5\text{-}HT_6$ and $5\text{-}HT_7$ receptors.

Bradykinin and Kallidin

As autacoids, bradykinin and kallidin:

- Increase vascular permeability
- Produce vasodilation
- Increase the synthesis of prostaglandins
- Cause edema and pain

Kinin Receptors

Kinin receptors are classified as kinin B_1 or kinin B_2. Kinin B_1 receptors, which are located in the aorta and mesenteric veins, respond to kinin agonists in the following order of potency:

des Arg^{10}-kallidin > des Arg^{10}-bradykinin
    > kallidin > [try(Mc^8)] bradykinin

Potential Therapeutic Uses

Preliminary data exist for a few potential uses of kinins in conditions such as male infertility due to **asthenozoospermia** and **oligospermia.** Kinins also have potential value in increasing the delivery of cancer chemotherapeutic agents beyond the blood–brain barrier.

Eicosanoids

All naturally occurring **prostaglandins** are derived through the **cyclization** of 20-carbon unsaturated fatty acids such as **arachidonic acid,** which in turn is synthesized from the essential fatty acid, **linoleic acid.**

Besides serving as a precursor for the synthesis of prostaglandins, arachidonic acid is also a precursor for the synthesis of prostacyclin, thromboxanes, and leukotrienes.

The prostaglandins are inactivated rapidly (half-life < 1 minute) by the pulmonary, hepatic, and renal vascular beds through the actions of prostaglandin dehydrogenase and prostaglandin reductase. **Prostacyclins** are also rapidly metabolized by prostaglandin dehydrogenase. **Thromboxane A_2** is hydrated in the blood to **thromboxane B_2.** The thromboxanes are metabolized extensively, and their metabolites appear in the urine.

The most important known effects of the prostaglandins and other eicosanoids are the **contraction** or **relaxation of smooth muscles.**

Smooth Muscles and Vascular Smooth Muscles

Prostaglandins E_2 and I_2 cause arteriolar dilation in the systemic and pulmonary vascular beds.

Respiratory Smooth Muscles

Prostaglandins E_1, E_2, and I_2 cause bronchodilation and oppose the actions of acetylcholine, histamine, and bradykinin.

Gastrointestinal Smooth Muscles

Prostaglandin E_2 contracts longitudinal but relaxes circular smooth muscles, whereas prostaglandin F_{2A} contracts both.

Reproductive Smooth Muscles

Prostaglandins E_1, E_2, and F_{2A} cause contraction of the pregnant and nonpregnant human uterus, and produce labor-like contractions. In contrast to **oxytocin,** this effect is possible in all stages of pregnancy.

In general, the constricting and relaxing effects of the eicosanoids on the smooth muscles are not mediated by means of the classic neurotransmitters such as acetylcholine, catecholamine, or histamine, as proved by the fact that they are not altered by antihistaminic substances, anticholinergic agents, or either alpha- or beta-adrenergic receptor-blocking agents.

Cardiovascular System

Prostaglandin E_2 and F_{2A} have positive inotropic effects and in general elicit increases in cardiac output.

Blood

Prostaglandin E_1 inhibits platelet aggregation, whereas thromboxane A_2 induces platelet aggregation. Prostaglandin A_2, E_1, and E_2 enhance erythropoiesis by augmenting the renal cortical release of **erythropoietin.**

Kidneys

Prostaglandins E_1, E_2, and I_2 increase renal blood flow and produce diuresis, natriuresis, and kaliuresis. Prostaglandins E_1 and E_2 antagonize the action of **antidiuretic hormone.**

Endocrine System

Various prostaglandins have the following effects in the endocrine system:

- Prostaglandins E_1 and F_{2A} stimulate the release of corticotropin.
- Prostaglandins E_1 and E_2 enhance the release of growth hormone.

- Prostaglandin F_{2A} increases the release of prolactin.
- Prostaglandin E_2 increases the release of luteinizing hormones.
- Prostaglandin F_{2A} reduces progesterone output and causes regression of the corpus luteum.

Metabolic Effects

Prostaglandin E_1 inhibits basal and catecholamine-stimulated lipolysis.

Nociception

Prostaglandins E_1 and E_2 bring about the sensation of pain by sensitizing the afferent nerve endings to noxious chemical and physical stimuli.

Inflammatory and Immune Responses

The prostaglandins are involved in both the genesis and manifestation of inflammation. Furthermore, prostaglandins are thought to regulate the functions of both B and T lymphocytes.

Central Nervous System

Prostaglandins E_1 and E_2 cause sedation.

Pyrexia

Prostaglandin E_1 precipitates fever when it is injected intracerebroventricularly.

Therapeutic Uses of Eicosanoids

Prostaglandins are mostly used as **abortifacients.** They may be administered by vaginal suppository (**Dino-** prostone), which contains prostaglandin E_2; by intramuscular injection (**carboprost** and **tromethamine**), which contains 15-methyl prostaglandin F_{2A}; or by intraamnionic administration (**dinoprost** and **tromethamine**), which contains prostaglandin F_{2A}. Other possible uses of prostaglandins may include the treatment of **ductus arteriosus** (prostaglandin E_1) to maintain patency and as a vasodilator (prostaglandin E_1) in the management of peripheral vascular diseases. High levels of prostaglandin F_{2A} may cause **dysmenorrhea,** as substances such as **indomethacin** and **ibuprofen** are effective in relieving these symptoms.

Aspirin, Prostaglandin, and Platelet Aggregation

Thromboxane A_2 is a potent vasoconstrictor and a stimulus to platelet aggregation; **prostacyclin,** on the other hand, is the principal cyclooxygenase product of the vascular endothelium and has the opposite effect on platelet function and vascular tone. **Aspirin** inhibits the arachidonic acid-induced platelet aggregation. It and other nonsteroidal antiinflammatory drugs block the biosynthesis of prostaglandins and thromboxane A_2 by inhibiting **cyclooxygenase.**

Indomethacin, Prostaglandin, and Ductus Arteriosus

The patency of the ductus arteriosus is maintained in part by a prostaglandin. **Indomethacin** induces constriction of the ductus during the neonatal period, whereas infusion of prostaglandin E_1 maintains its patency.

CHAPTER 33

Hormones and Neurotransmitters Activating the Cellular Signal Transduction System

A large number of neurotransmitters, hormones, and pharmacologic substances are responsible for eliciting the integrated responses of target cells by first interacting with plasma membrane receptors. Of these, the **cyclic adenosine monophosphate** (cAMP) **cascade** is the most ubiquitous and of greatest importance for the purposes of pharmacotherapy. Most of these substances trigger cellular **signal transduction mechanisms** by activating guanosine monophosphate(G)-protein-coupled receptors.

G-Protein-Coupled Receptors

Receptor-G Protein Interaction

Adenylate cyclase is activated by G-protein-coupled receptors such as the beta$_2$-adrenergic receptors. When complexed with a G protein, the receptor often has a higher affinity for its agonist. When the G protein forms a complex with an agonist-occupied receptor, the dissociation of guanosine diphosphate (GDP) and the binding of guanosine triphosphate (GTP) in the G-protein alpha subunit occur more rapidly. Receptors form complexes with heteroisomeric GTP-binding proteins that consist of alpha, beta, and gamma subunits.

Receptor Desensitization

Prolonged exposure to the agonists of several G-protein-coupled receptors (e.g., adrenergic receptors, muscarinic receptors, and tachykinin) causes desensitization that is characterized by the need for increased concentration of agonists in order to produce half-maximal stimulation of adenylate cyclase.

Protein Kinase, Phosphorylation, and Receptor Regulation

Two different kinases are involved in phosphorylating beta-adrenergic receptors. **Protein kinase A** is positively regulated by cAMP and is stimulated by substances that activate adenylate cyclase. **Beta adrenergic receptor kinase** (BARK) is related functionally to rhodopsin kinase and may be important for regulating neural transmission. A cytosolic protein, **beta-arrestin,** interacts with the BARK-phosphorylated receptors and disrupts the activation of G$_3$ by the beta receptor.

Redistribution of Receptors

Receptors may be regulated by two different processes: (1) **receptor sequestration,** which represents the rapid (within minutes) and reversible removal of functional receptors from the plasma membrane, and (2) **receptor down-regulation,** which occurs slowly (over hours) and may result in a significant and irreversible loss of the receptors.

Receptors for Physiologic Regulatory Molecules

Following are descriptions of several substances that alter the integrity of the G-protein receptors.

Cholera Toxin - **Choleragen,** the secretory product of *Vibrio cholerae,* can persistently activate adenylate cyclase by catalyzing the transfer of the adenosine diphosphate (ADP)–ribose moiety of nicotinamide adenosine dinucleotide (NAD$^+$) to G$_{sa}$.

Pertussis Toxin - The secretory product of *Bordetella pertussis* interferes with the ability of agonists to inhibit adenylate cyclase. It catalyzes the transfer of the ADP-ribose moiety of NAD^+ to a cysteine residue close to the carboxy terminus of G_{ia}.

Forskolin - Forskolin, which is isolated from *Coleus forskohlii,* stimulates adenylate cyclase.

Calmodulin - Calcium plays a major role in regulating cyclic nucleotide metabolism, and its effects show tissue specificity. In physiologic ranges, calcium activates adenylate cyclase in the brain. This calcium-mediated activation of adenylate cyclase is thought to take place through the binding of calcium to calmodulin, a low-molecular-weight calcium-binding protein homologous to skeletal muscle **troponin C.**

Cyclic Nucleotides

Synthesis of Cyclic Nucleotides

The interaction of an agonist such as epinephrine with its receptor sites results in the synthesis and accumulation of cAMP. This then activates a cAMP-dependent protein kinase, which mediates the catalytic transfer of a gamma phosphate from ATP to a protein that serves as the final substrate underlying the physiologic effects of the agonist that had initially interacted with the receptor sites.

Physiologic Substances and the Cyclic Nucleotides

Calcitonin - The concentration of calcitonin in the plasma increases in the presence of hypercalcemia. Therefore, calcitonin is effective in combating hypercalcemia in patients with vitamin D intoxication and hyperparathyroidism. Calcitonin does not have an antiparathyroid effect and does not block the activation of adenylate cyclase by parathyroid hormone.

Adrenocorticotropic Hormone - Adrenocorticotropic hormone (ACTH; corticotropin) stimulates the adrenal gland to secrete the glucocorticoids and mineralocorticoids. ACTH is thought to bring about these effects by enhancing the cAMP concentration.

Antidiuretic Hormone - The antidiuretic hormone activates adenylate cyclase at the basolateral membrane, thus increasing the cAMP level, which in turn enhances the permeability of the luminal cell surface to water.

Glucagon and Insulin - The hyperglycemic (antiinsulin) effect of epinephrine and glucagon is mediated by cAMP. Insulin has been shown to inhibit the activity of adenylate cyclase and to stimulate the activity of phosphodiesterase.

Gonadotropins - Luteinizing hormones and follicle-stimulating hormone are responsible for increasing testicular growth, spermatogenesis, and steroidogenesis. All of these effects are mediated by cyclic nucleotides.

Trophic Hormones - Melanocyte-stimulating hormone, thyrotropin-releasing hormone, and thyroid-stimulating hormone use cAMP as a second messenger, and their effect is mediated by this mechanism.

Drugs Used in the Treatment of Asthma

Cyclic Adenosine Monophosphate and Bronchial Asthma

Cyclic adenosine monophosphate prevents bronchial smooth muscle contraction, promotes bronchial smooth muscle relaxation, and inhibits the release of mediators. The metabolism of cAMP takes place according to the following scheme:

$$ATP \xrightarrow{\text{Adenylate cyclase}} cAMP \xrightarrow{\text{Phosphodiesterase}} 5' \, AMP$$

Agents that stimulate the activity of adenylate cyclase (beta$_2$ agonists), inhibit the activity of phosphodiesterase (aminophylline), or enhance the effects of beta$_2$ agonists on their receptor sites (corticosteroids) are extremely useful **antiasthmatic agents.** Conversely, substances that block the beta-adrenergic receptor site (propranolol) or that stimulate either the cholinergic receptor sites (cholinomimetic agents) or the alpha-adrenergic receptor site (prostaglandin F_{2A}) cause **bronchoconstriction.** Furthermore, the muscarinic cholinergic receptor antagonists (ipratropium bromide) are potential **bronchodilators.**

CHAPTER 34

Calcium and Calcium Channel Blocking Agents

Many hormones, neurotransmitters, and autacoids exert their actions by altering phosphoinositide metabolism, increasing the concentration of ionized calcium in the cytosol of their target cells, and stimulating the turnover rate of phosphatidylinositol 4,5-bisphosphate (PIP_2).

Voltage-Activated and Receptor-Operated Calcium Channels

Under normal conditions, the extracellular concentration of calcium is in the millimolar range (10^{-3} M), whereas its intracellular concentration is less than 10^{-7} M. The cytoplasmic concentration of calcium is increased through the actions of **receptor-operated channels, voltage-activated channels,** or **ionic pumps.** In addition, calcium can be released from internal stores.

There are two types of voltage-activated channels:

1. **Low-voltage-activated channels** or low-threshold channels, which are also termed *T-type channels*
2. **High-voltage-activated channels,** which are further subdivided into L-type, N-type, and P-type channels

Calcium and Transmitter Release

The secretion of neurotransmitters and neurohormone is usually triggered by a rise in the intracellular calcium concentration. However, the release of **acetylcholine** from the Schwann cells and **renin** from the juxtaglomerular apparatus is triggered by a fall in the intracellular calcium level.

Unlike skeletal muscles, which contain endogenous stores of calcium ions, both cardiac muscle and vascular smooth muscle require extracellular calcium for contractile function. Therefore, cardiac muscle and vascular smooth muscle are subject to regulation by **calcium antagonists** or **calcium entry blockers,** which are used in the treatment of **hypertension, Raynaud's disease, Prinzmetal's angina,** and **migraine syndromes.**

Agents Affecting Calcium Movements

When calcium homeostasis fails, as occurs in the presence of **anoxia,** cell viability is threatened by the uncontrolled influx of calcium through the plasma membrane or by the massive release of calcium from intracellular binding and sequestration sites. Agents that affect calcium movements consist of **calcium entry blockers** and **calcium antagonists.**

Calcium Entry Blockers

Calcium entry blockers include agents that are **selective for slow calcium channels** in the myocardium (slow channel blockers) and consist of the following categories of substances:

Phenylalkylamines — verapamil, gallopamil, anipamil, desmethoxyverapamil, emopamil, falipamil, and ronipamil

Dihydropyridines — nifedipine, nicardipine, niludipine, nimodipine, nisoldipine, nitrendipine, ryosidine, amlodipine, azodipine, dazodipine, felodipine, flordipine, iodipine, isrodipine, mesudipine, oxodipine, and riodipine

Benzothiazepines — diltiazem

Calcium Agonists

Three groups of agents serve as calcium agonists (facilitators), depending on their site of action: Agents that act at the **plasma membrane** consist of the **dihydropyridines.** Agents that act on the **sacroplasmic reticulum** include inositol 1,4,5-triphosphate and caffeine. The last group consists of the **ionophores** (ionomycin).

Calcium Entry Blockers and Their Use in Various Disorders

Hypertension

Verapamil, nifedipine, and **diltiazem** lower blood pressure with an efficacy comparable to that achieved by other commonly used agents. Their specific effects on the cardiovascular system are listed in ■ **Table 34-1** ■.

The IV administration of diltiazem or verapamil or the oral or sublingual administration of nifedipine is effective in managing hypertensive emergencies.

Myocardial Infarction

Heart failure is associated with changes in the intracellular calcium levels. The rationale for using calcium entry blockers in preventing the secondary complications of myocardial infarction stems from the fact that these agents reduce systemic vascular resistance, afterload, myocardial contractility, blood pressure, and oxygen consumption. Despite these effects, the efficacy of calcium entry blockers in preventing the secondary complications of myocardial infarction or their usefulness in the context of cerebrovascular diseases such as aneurysmal subarachnoid hemorrhage needs to be established.

Angina

Beta-adrenergic blocking agents are effective for the prophylactic therapy of **exertional angina pectoris** by reducing heart rate and the force of myocardial contraction. Verapamil, nifedipine, and diltiazem are also effective for the prophylactic treatment of stable exertional angina. The combination therapy with beta blockers and calcium entry blockers is well tolerated, effective, and safe.

Psychiatric Disorders

Verapamil has been used in the treatment of mania, depression, maintenance control of manic depression, and schizophrenia. In addition, it has been used in the management of premenstrual syndrome, stuttering, and intoxication with phencyclidine.

Cerebrovascular Disorders

Among the various types of calcium entry blockers, **flunarizine** has proved to be the most effective in the prophylaxis of **migraine.** It has also been shown to be beneficial in protecting brain cells against **hypoxia** and in preventing the constriction of cerebrovascular smooth muscle cells. Moreover, it has been shown to be effective in the treatment of **epilepsy** and **hemiplegia.**

Parkinson's Disease

Calcium entry blockers may induce **extrapyramidal symptoms** and aggravate parkinsonism.

Drug Interactions and Calcium Entry Blockers

Following are some of the drug interactions seen with either specific calcium entry blockers or these agents in general:

- Verapamil inhibits several oxidative routes of hepatic metabolism.
- Verapamil and diltiazem decrease the clearance of **theophylline** and increase its half-life.
- Calcium channel blockers increase the toxicity of **lithium,** which has calcium antagonist effects itself.
- Calcium channel blockers potentiate the negative inotropic effects of type Ia antiarrhythmic agents.
- Verapamil increases the plasma concentration of **digitoxin.**
- Calcium entry blockers potentiate the hypotensive effects of **prazocin.**
- Calcium entry blockers increase the plasma concentration of **carbamazepine.**
- Calcium entry blockers decrease the clearance of **cyclosporine.**
- Calcium entry blockers impair myocardial conduction when given with **enflurane** and precipitate pronounced hypotension when given with **halothane.**

■ **Table 34-1** ■ Effects of Calcium Entry Blockers on the Cardiovascular System

Drugs	Heart Rate	Atrioventricular Nodal Conduction	Myocardial Contractility	Arteriolar Vasodilation
Verapamil	No change	Greatly decreased	Moderately decreased	Moderately increased
Nifedipine	Increased	—	No change	Greatly increased
Diltiazem	Decreased	Moderately decreased	Decreased	Increased

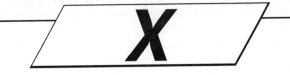

X

Antimicrobial Chemotherapy and Therapy of Tuberculosis and Parasitic Diseases

CHAPTER 35

Antimicrobial Chemotherapy

General Pharmacodynamics of Chemotherapeutic Agents

The effects of antimicrobial agents are brought about by four different mechanisms:

1. Inhibition of **cell wall synthesis** — for example, penicillins, cephalosporins, bacitracin, cycloserine, and vancomycin ■ **Fig. 35-1** ■
2. Inhibition of the functions of **cellular membranes** — for example, amphotericin B, colistin, nystatin, and polymyxin ■ **Fig. 35-2** ■
3. Inhibition of **nucleic acid synthesis** (antimetabolites) — for example, sulfonamides, trimethoprim, nalidixic acid, rifampin, and pyrimethamine See ■ **Fig. 35-1** ■
4. Inhibition of **protein synthesis** — for example, chloramphenicol, erythromycins, tetracyclines, and aminoglycosides See ■ **Fig. 35-2** ■

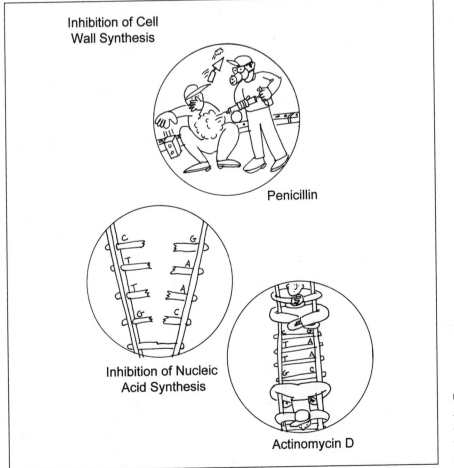

Inhibition of Cell Wall Synthesis

Penicillin

Inhibition of Nucleic Acid Synthesis

Actinomycin D

■ **Fig. 35-1** ■
Antibiotics inhibiting the construction of the cell wall or the synthesis of nucleic acid.

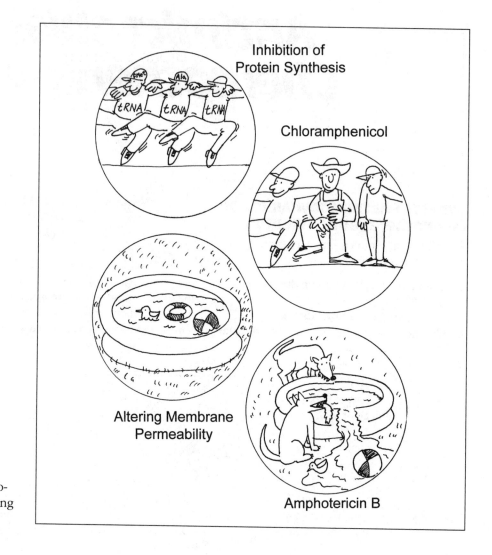

Inhibition of
Protein Synthesis

Chloramphenicol

Altering Membrane
Permeability

Amphotericin B

■ **Fig. 35-2** ■
Antibiotics inhibiting protein synthesis or damaging cellular membrane.

Actions and Spectrum of Activity

When exerting their effects, antimicrobial agents either kill the cells (**bactericidals** such as penicillin) or **inhibit microbial replication (bacteriostatics** such as the sulfonamides). The antimicrobial agents may also have either a narrow or broad spectrum of activity during which they can inhibit both gram-positive and gram-negative bacteria (e.g., the tetracyclines). ■ **Fig. 35-3** ■

Antibiotic Synergism and Antagonism

In the eradication of infectious diseases, antibiotics are often used in combinations that must be selected carefully. Not all antibiotics have synergistic effects, and they may have deleterious antagonistic effects. For example, penicillin, streptomycin, bacitracin, and the polymyxins have synergistic effects and may be used together in certain combinations. On the other hand, chloramphenicol, the tetracyclines, erythromycin, and the sulfonamides are seldom used in combination. In fact, some of these agents, such as chloramphenicol, can even oppose the bacterial actions of the penicillins or aminoglycosides. See ■ **Fig. 35-3** ■

The Drugs

The selection of antibiotics is based on the pattern of sensitivity of the infecting organism or organisms. In addition, other factors must be taken into serious consideration: the patient's age, the status of the patient's liver to metabolize the drugs, the status of the patient's kidney to excrete the drug or its metabolites, any genetic disorders that could alter the pharmacokinetics of the drugs, and the history of drug allergy, among others.

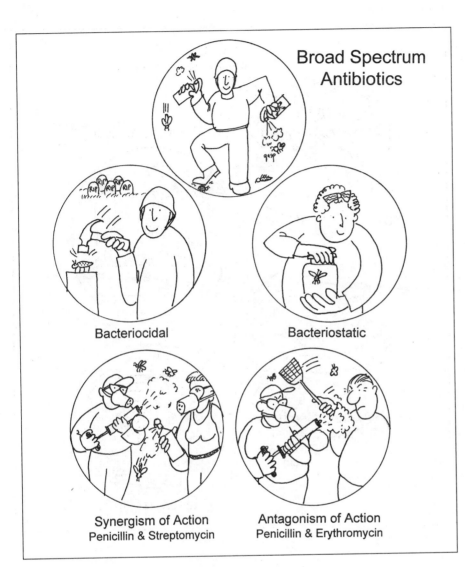

Broad Spectrum Antibiotics

Bacteriocidal

Bacteriostatic

Synergism of Action
Penicillin & Streptomycin

Antagonism of Action
Penicillin & Erythromycin

■ Fig. 35-3 ■
Nature of actions and
reactions of antibiotics.

Complications of Antimicrobial Therapy

The complications of therapy with antibiotics are bacterial resistance to the drugs, the emergence of superinfections, and the appearance of toxic reactions.

Sulfonamides and Trimethoprim-Sulfamethoxazole

Mechanism of Action - By competing with para-aminobenzoic acid (PABA), the sulfonamides inhibit the synthesis of folic acid, which is essential for the production of purines by bacteria and their ultimate synthesis of nucleic acids. They are also incorporated into folic acid. ■ **Fig. 35-4** ■

Toxicities - Many of the adverse reactions seen with sulfonamides are due to **hypersensitivity reactions,** which include dermatitis, leukopenia, hemolytic ane-

mia, and drug fever. **Stevens-Johnson syndrome** is a very severe, but rare, hypersensitivity reaction that occurs only with some of the long-acting sulfonamide preparations.

Renal lesions may be due to the precipitation of sulfonamides and their acetyl derivatives in the urinary tract. **Renal damage** may also be attributable to a direct toxic effect of sulfonamides on the kidney tubules.

Sulfonamides may cause **jaundice** and **kernicterus** in newborns. This is due to the displacement of **bilirubin** from protein-binding sites. Therefore, sulfonamides should not be used during pregnancy.

Trimethoprim-Sulfamethoxazole

The combination of trimethoprim and sulfamethoxazole (usually five parts sulfamethoxazole to one part trimethoprim) interferes with the **synthesis of active folic acid** by means of two separate reactions. In the

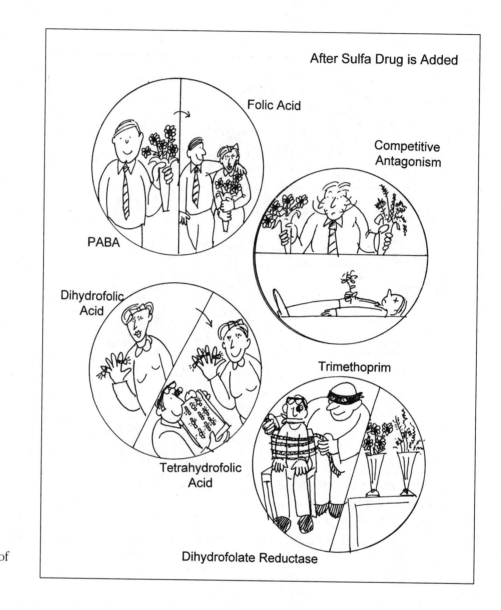

■ **Fig. 35-4** ■
Mechanisms of action of sulfonamides.

first, sulfonamides compete with PABA and prevent its conversion to dihydrofolic acid. In the second, trimethoprim, by inhibiting the activity of **dihydrofolic acid reductase,** prevents the conversion of dihydrofolic acid into tetrahydrofolic acid, which is necessary for the synthesis of DNA. These reactions ■ **Figs. 35-4 and 35-5** ■ are summarized as follows:

p-Aminobenzoic acid (PABA)
↓   ⊬ Sulfonamides
Dihydrofolic acid
↓   ⊬ Trimethoprim
Tetrahydrofolic acid
↓
Deoxyuridylate ⟶ Thymidylate
↓
DNA

These drug combinations have the following **therapeutic advantages:**

■ They cause synergistic antibacterial effects.
■ They have bactericidal activity.
■ The emergence of bacterial resistance is decreased.
■ The spectrum of antibacterial activity is enhanced.
■ Toxicity is reduced.

Folic acid deficiency may occur following prolonged usage of **methotrexate** or in patients with preexisting folic acid deficiency. **Folinic acid** may be administered to overcome the folic-acid deficiency-related megaloblastic anemia.

Clinical Uses - Orally administered trimethoprim is used in the treatment of chronic recurring urinary tract infection. Oral forms of trimethoprim-sulfamethoxazole

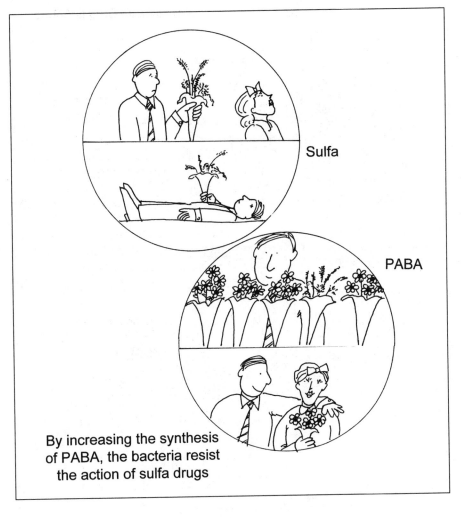

By increasing the synthesis
of PABA, the bacteria resist
the action of sulfa drugs

Sulfa

PABA

■ Fig. 35-5 ■
Development of resistance
to sulfonamides.

are used in *Shigella* and some *Salmonella* infections, particularly when they are resistant to ampicillin and chloramphenicol.

The Quinolones

The quinolones include **nalidix acid** (NegGram), **cinoxacin** (Cinobac), **norfloxacin** (Noroxin), and **ciprofloxacin** (Cipro). Other members of the quinolone family are **perfloxacin, ofloxacin, enoxacin,** and **fleroxacin.**

Mechanism of Action - The bacterial enzyme **DNA gryrase** is responsible for the continuous introduction of negative supercoils into DNA, and the quinolones inhibit this gyrase-mediated DNA supercoiling.

Adverse Effects - The quinolones and fluoroquinolones may produce **arthropathy,** and hence should not be used in prepubertal children or pregnant women.

Clinical Uses - **Nalidix acid** and **cinoxacin** are useful only for treating urinary tract infections. **Ciprofloxacin** is useful for both urinary tract infections and prostatitis.

Urinary Tract Antiseptics

Methenamine mandelate (Mandelamine) decomposes in solution to generate **formaldehyde,** which in a concentration of 20 μg/ml inhibits all bacteria-causing urinary tract infections. Urea-splitting microorganisms (*Proteus* species) raise the pH of the urine and hence inhibit the release of formaldehyde and the action of methenamine. On the other hand, acidification of the urine enhances the antibacterial action of methenamine.

Nitrofurantoin (Furadantin) may cause **neuropathies** when used for a long period and in patients with impaired renal functions.

Phenazopyridine hydrochloride (Pyridium) is not an antiseptic but a **urinary tract analgesic** and may be used in the management of dysuria, burning, and urgency.

Penicillins and Their Newer Derivatives

Penicillin is an organic acid, which is commonly supplied as sodium and potassium salts. Penicillin V (Pen Vee K and V-Cillin K) and phenethicillin (Syncillin and Maxipen) are different from penicillin G (Benzylpenicillin) in that they are more acid resistant. In addition to the broad-spectrum penicillins such as ampicillin and amoxicillin, there is a newer group of anti-*Pseudomonas* penicillins that are effective against gram-negative bacilli. These agents include carbenicillin, ticarcillin, azlocillin, and piperacillin. The latter two agents are also useful against *Klebsiella pneumoniae* and *Bacteroides fragilis*. ■ **Fig. 35-6** ■

The **penicillinase-resistant penicillins** are oxacillin, cloxacillin, dicloxacillin, methicillin, and nafcillin. These agents are the drugs of choice for treating infections caused by penicillinase-producing *Staphylococci aureus*.

Mechanism of Action - Penicillins achieve their effect by inhibiting formation of cell walls, and hence are bactericidal. Penicillin binds to cellular receptors, now identified as **transpeptidation enzymes,** and by binding to and inhibiting the transpeptidation reactions, the synthesis of cell wall **peptidoglycan** is interrupted. In addition, penicillin removes or inactivates an inhibitor of the lytic enzymes (**autolysin**), resulting in the lysis of microorganisms in an isotonic environment. In general, penicillins are more active against **gram-positive organisms.** See ■ **Fig. 35-1** ■

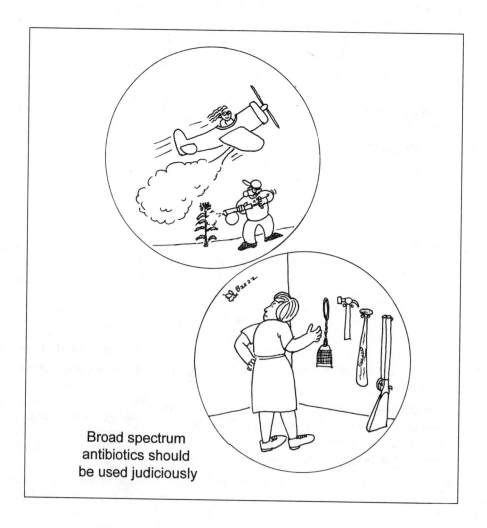

■ **Fig. 35-6** ■

Proper selection of antibiotics.

Broad spectrum antibiotics should be used judiciously

Therapeutic Applications - Penicillin G may be used either actively or prophylactically for the following clinical settings:

- Streptococcal infections
- Pneumococcal infections
- Staphylococcal infections (generally resistant, to penicillin G)
- Meningococcal disease
- Gonococcal infections
- Syphilis
- Actinomycosis, anthrax, and gas gangrene

Adverse Effects - Penicillins, which are the safest of antibiotics, produce few direct toxic reactions, and most of the serious side effects are **hypersensitivity reactions.**

The **broad-spectrum penicillins,** such as **ampicillin** and **amoxicillin,** may cause GI irritation. Occasionally the overgrowth of staphylococci, *Pseudomonas, Proteus,* or yeasts may be responsible for causing **enteritis.** Methicillin and nafcillin may precipitate **granulocytopenia,** and methicillin has been known to cause **nephritis.** Carbenicillin may cause **hypokalemic alkalosis.**

Antipseudomonal Penicillins

Carbenicillin cures serious infections caused by *Pseudomonas* species and *Proteus* strains resistant to ampicillin.

Cephalosporins

Like the penicillins, cephalosporins exert their effects by inhibiting the formation of cell walls in the bacteria. Clinical resistance to some of the second- and third-generation cephalosporins has been reported. These agents are resistant to **penicillinase-producing organisms.**

Cephalexin, cefaclor, cefadroxil, and cephradine are absorbed well from the GI tract and thus are given orally. Cephaloridine, cephalothin, cephapirin, cefoxitin, cefotaxime, cefamandole, and cefazolin are poorly absorbed from the GI tract and must be given parenterally. Because the cephalosporins have short half-lives, they must be administered frequently. First- and second-generation (but not third-generation) cephalosporins do not readily penetrate the CNS and therefore are not effective for the treatment of meningitis. The cephalosporins are eliminated by **glomerular filtration** and **active tubular secretion,** which are blocked by **probenecid.** The acetylated derivatives of cephalosporins, such as cephalothin and cephapirin, are metabolized in the liver to inactive metabolites.

Clinical Uses - The cephalosporins, often in combination with aminoglycoside antibiotics, are used in suspected cases of bacteremia due to *Staphylococcus, Klebsiella,* coliform bacteria, *Proteus,* or *Pseudomonas* infection.

Adverse Effects - The adverse reactions caused by cephalosporins resemble those named for penicillin and include injection-site complications, phlebitis following IV administration, hypersensitivity reactions, and rare anaphylactoid shock. Infrequently, nephrotoxicity does occur with some cephalosporins.

Aminoglycoside Antibiotics

Aminoglycosides are bactericidal and **inhibit protein synthesis** in susceptible microorganisms. They exert this effect by (1) interfering with the initiation complex of peptide formation, (2) inducing misreading of the code on the messenger RNA template, which causes the incorporation of inappropriate amino acid into peptide, and (3) rupturing the polysomes into monosomes, which become nonfunctional.

The aminoglycosides are poorly absorbed from the GI tract and for this reason are administered intramuscularly.

The most serious toxic reactions following aminoglycoside therapy are **cochlear damage** and **vestibular impairment,** which lead to vertigo and disturb the ability to maintain postural equilibrium. Aminoglycosides given during pregnancy cause **deafness** in the newborn. **Nephrotoxicity** and reversible neuromuscular blockade causing respiratory paralysis have also been seen following the use of high doses.

Erythromycin

Erythromycin (Erythrocin, Ilotycin), as a penicillin alternative, is a medium- to broad-spectrum antibiotic.

Erythromycin exerts its effect by binding to 23S ribosomal RNA on the 50S ribosomal subunit, and this inhibits protein synthesis. Aminoactyl translocation reactions and elongation of the peptide chain are then blocked. See ■ **Fig. 35-2** ■

Erythromycin and especially erythromycin estolate can cause **cholestatic hepatitis.**

Chloramphenicol

Chloramphenicol (Chloromycetin) has a broad spectrum of bacteriostatic activity for many bacteria, including *Rickettsia.* It is the preferred drug in the treatment of *Salmonella* infection (e.g., typhoid fever); *Haemophilus influenzae,* meningitis, laryngotracheitis, or pneumonia not responding to ampicillin; *Bacteroides* infections; meningococcal infections in patients allergic to penicillin; and *Rickettsia* infections.

Chloramphenicol exerts its effects by binding to 50S ribosomal subunits and thus inhibiting bacterial protein synthesis, by preventing peptide-bond formation, and by inhibiting the synthesis of mitochondrial proteins in the host. See ■ **Fig. 35-2** ■

Chloramphenicol causes both dose-dependent and dose-independent hematologic reactions. Fatal **aplastic anemia** occurs in genetically susceptible patients taking chloramphenicol on a long-term basis. Reversible and dose-dependent disturbances of **hemopoiesis** can also arise and are characterized by the altered maturation of red blood cells, vacuolated and nucleated red blood cell in the marrow, and reticulocytopenia.

Newborn infants are deficient in **glucuronyl transferase.** Thus, doses of chloramphenicol for newborns should not exceed 50 mg/kg per day. Large doses will precipitate **gray baby syndrome,** characterized by vomiting, hypothermia, gray skin tone, and shock.

Tetracyclines

Tetracyclines, which are bacteriostatic, have the broadest spectrum of activity and are effective against infections with gram-positive and gram-negative bacteria, *Rickettsia,* mycoplasma, amoeba, and *Chlamydia.*

Tetracyclines enter bacterial cells by both passive diffusion and active transport, and then they accumulate intracellularly. This does not occur in mammalian cells. The tetracyclines bind to the 30S subunit of the bacterial ribosome in such a way that the binding of the aminoacyl-transfer RNA to the acceptor site on the messenger RNA ribosome complex is blocked.

The absorption of tetracyclines is impaired by **divalent cations** (calcium, magnesium, and ferrous iron), by aluminum, and by extremely alkaline pHs.

Tetracyclines are effective in the treatment of Rocky Mountain spotted fever, murine typhus, recrudescent epidemic typhus, scrub typhus, Q fever, lymphogranuloma venereum, psittacosis, tularemia, brucellosis, gonorrhea, certain urinary tract infections, granuloma inguinale, chancroid, syphilis, and diseases due to *Bacteroides* and *Clostridium.*

Tetracyclines have been known to cause hepatic necrosis, especially when given in large IV doses or when taken by pregnant women or patients with pre-existing liver impairment. Tetracycline preparations whose potency has expired can cause **renal tubular acidosis.** With the exception of doxycycline, tetracyclines accumulate in patients with renal impairment. Tetracyclines also produce **nitrogen retention,** especially when given with diuretics. The systemic administration of **demeclocycline** elicits **photosensitization** to ultraviolet light or sunlight. **Minocycline** causes vertigo and dizziness. Tetracyclines bind to calcium and then become deposited in bone, causing damage to developing bone and teeth. The IV administration of tetracyclines has been observed to cause **venous thrombosis.**

Polypeptide Antibiotics

Bacitracin - Bacitracin (Baciquent), which inhibits cell wall synthesis, is active against gram-positive bacteria.

Polymyxins - The polymyxins consist of polymyxin B (Aerosporin) and polymyxin E, or colisten (Coly-Mycin). These agents, which are bactericidal, are effective in the management of gram-negative bacteria infections, especially *Pseudomonas.*

CHAPTER 36

Antifungal Agents

Fungal Diseases

The fungal diseases are histoplasmosis, coccidiodomycosis, blastomycosis, paracoccidiodomycosis, cryptococcosis, sporotrichosis, candidiasis, aspergillosis, and mucormycosis.

Antifungal Agents

The antifungal agents consist of either topical or systemic medications. The **systemic antifungal agents** include:

- Amphotericin B
- Flucytosine
- Ketoconazole
- Griseofulvin
- Nystatin

Amphotericin B

Amphotericin B (Fungizone), which is ineffective in ridding infections caused by bacteria, *Rickettsia,* or viruses, is either fungicidal or fungistatic, depending on the drug concentration used or the sensitivity of the particular fungus. Numerous pathogenic yeasts (*Cryptococcus neoformans*), pathogenic yeastlike organisms (*Monilia*), dimorphic fungi (*Blastomyces*), filamentous fungi (*Cladosporosium*), and other fungi are highly sensitive to amphotericin B. Furthermore, the antifungal actions of amphotericin B are enhanced by **flucytosine, minocycline,** or **rifampin,** agents otherwise devoid of antifungal activity.

Amphotericin B imposes its antifungal effects by binding to the **sterol moiety** of the membrane and damaging its structural and functional integrity. See **■ Fig. 35-2 ■**

Amphotericin B is **nephrotoxic** in most patients and often causes a permanent reduction in glomerular filtration rate. Furthermore, **hypokalemia** may occur, requiring the oral administration of potassium chloride.

Amphotericin B has been used intrathecally in patients with **coccidiodal** or **cryptococcal meningitis.** The side effects associated with this route of administration are headache, paresthesia, nerve palsy, and visual impairment. To treat **coccidiodial arthritis,** amphotericin B may be injected intraarticularly.

Flucytosine

Flucytosine (Ancobon) possesses clinically useful activity against *C. neoformans, Candida* species, *Torulopsis glabrata,* and the agents of chromomycosis. Susceptible fungi deaminate flucytosine to **5-fluorouracil,** which becomes an antimetabolite. Flucytosine, which is excreted by the kidney, should be used cautiously in renal impairment. Flucytosine is a bone marrow depressant. Flucytosine is used in combination with amphotericin B.

Ketoconazole

Ketoconazole (Nizoral) has a broad therapeutic potential for a number of superficial and systemic fungal infections. Ketoconazole dissolves in an acidic media; therefore, antacids or histamine$_2$-receptor-blocking agents reduce its effectiveness. Ketoconazole can cause GI disturbances.

Griseofulvin

Griseofulvin (Fulvicin and Grisactin) is a fungistatic agent effective against various **dermatophytes,** including *Microsporum, Epidermophyton,* and *Trichophyton,* that produce diseases of the skin, hair, and nails. It exerts its effect by inhibiting **fungal mitosis.**

Nystatin

Nystatin (Mycostatin) is poorly absorbed from the GI tract. It is both fungistatic and fungicidal but has no effect on bacteria, viruses, or protozoa. It exerts its effect by binding to the sterol moiety and hence damaging the fungal membrane. See **■ Fig. 35-2 ■** It is used primarily as a topical agent to treat candidal infections of the skin and mucous membrane (paronychia, vaginitis, and stomatitis) and causes no major toxicities.

CHAPTER 37

Therapy of Helminthic, Protozoal, and Mycobacterial Diseases

The pharmacology of the most often used anti-helminthics is summarized in ■ **Table 37-1** ■.

Protozoal Infections

Amebiasis

Treatment of the Asymptomatic Carrier - Effective drugs for treating the asymptomatic carrier are the 8-hydroxyquinolone derivatives, such as **iodoquinol** (the preferred drug) and **diloxanide furoate** (an alternative drug).

Treatment of Acute Dysentery - **Dehydroemetine** is given for 5 days and effects rapid relief of the symptoms of acute amebic dysentery. The patient is then switched to **metronidazole.** If the response to metronidazole is not satisfactory, dehydroemetine plus tetracycline or dehydroemetine plus paromomycin are given along with the metronidazole.

Treatment of Amebic Hepatitis and Abscess - Amebic hepatitis and abscess are best treated with metronidazole. Dehydroemetine or chlorquine can serve as alternate drugs.

Malaria
The selected pharmacologic properties of the most often used antimalarial agents are listed in ■ **Table 37-2** ■.

Leishmaniasis
Agents effective in the treatment of leishmaniasis are the pentavalent antimonials, **pentamidine,** amphotericin B (Fungizone), sodium stibogluconate (Sb³), dehydroemetine resinate (Mebadin), and metronidazole (Flagyl).

Trypanosomiasis
Agents effective in the treatment of trypanosomiasis are the **aromatic diamidines** (pentamidine, stil-bamidine, and propamidine). **Pentamidine** is the preferred drug for the prevention and early treatment of *Trypanosoma gambiense* infections; however, it cannot penetrate the CNS. **Melarsoprol** is the drug recommended for *T. gambiense* infections that do not respond to pentamidine or for managing the late meningoencephalitic stages of infection. It does reach the CNS. **Nifurtimox** (Lampit) is the drug of choice for treating the acute form of Chagas' disease. **Suramin** (Naphuride) is effective only in the therapy for African sleeping sickness.

Toxoplasmosis
Pyrimethamine, in combination with sulfadiazine, is the preferred treatment for *Toxoplasma gondii* infection. Corticosteroids are added to the therapeutic regimen in patients with severe chorioretinitis.

Mycobacterial Diseases

Tuberculosis
The pharmacologic properties of the drugs most often used to treat tuberculosis are summarized in ■ **Table 37-3** ■.

Leprosy
Dapsone and **sulfoxone** sodium are the most useful and effective agents currently available. With adequate precautions and appropriate doses, sulfones may be used safely for years. Nevertheless, side effects such as anorexia, nervousness, insomnia, blurred vision, paresthesia, and peripheral neuropathy do occur. **Hemolysis** is common, especially in patients with glucose-6-phosphate dehydrogenase deficiency.

■ Table 37-1 ■ Pharmacology of the Antihelminthics

Antihelminthics	Properties
Pyrantel pamoate (Antiminth)	Pyrantel is poorly absorbed from the GI tract, and most (80%) is eliminated in the feces. It is a drug of choice in ascariasis and enterobiasis. Pyrantel is a depolarizing neuromuscular blocking agent causing spastic paralysis of the hookworm, pinworm, and roundworm.
Mebendazole (Vermox)	Mebendazole exerts its broad-spectrum antihelminthic property by irreversibly inhibiting glucose uptake. It is effective against ascariasis, capillariasis, enterobiasis, and trichuriasis.
Pyrvinium pamoate (Vanquin, Povan)	Pyrvinium is not absorbed from the GI tract. It is thought to exert its effects by inhibiting oxygen uptake and hence inhibiting respiration in nematodes.
Piperazine citrate (Antepar)	Piperazine is absorbed from the GI tract. Since lethal doses cause convulsions, it should not be used in patients with epilepsy. It exerts its antihelminthic effects by causing flacid paralysis of muscle, resulting in expulsion of the worm.
Thiabendazole (Mintezol)	Thiabendazole is absorbed rapidly from the GI tract. It is metabolized by hydroxylation and conjugation with glucuronic acid. The commonly occurring side effects are anorexia, nausea, and dizziness. It should be used with caution in patients with decreased hepatic function. The mechanism of action of thiabendazole is not known. However, it selectively inhibits fumarate reductase and prevents the embryonic development of *Ascaris* eggs in vitro.
Niclosamide (Yomesan)	Niclosamide, which is not absorbed from the GI tract, is the safest effective drug in cestode infestations. It inhibits anerobic metabolism and glucose intake in *Taenia solium*, against which it is a highly effective drug. Since lethal doses of niclosamide in adult worms do not destroy the ova, purgation 1–2 h after niclosamide is essential, or the risk of cysticercosis is likely.
Metrifonate (Bilarcil)	Metrifonate is an organophosphorus-inhibiting cholinesterase in *Schistosoma haematobium*. Since the plasma cholinesterase in the host is similarly inhibited, depolarizing neuromuscular blocking agents, other cholinesterase inhibitors, and agents metabolized by plasma cholinesterase should not be administered with metrifonate.
Praziquantel (Biltricide, Droncit)	Praziquantel, which is absorbed orally, is effective against all schistosomes. It dislodges the worm in the intestine and subjects the tegmen to proteolysis. It is also effective against cestodes.
Oxamniquine (Vansil)	Oxamniquine, which is absorbed following oral administration, is very effective only in *Schistosoma mansoni*. Following treatment, the *S. mansoni* shifts from the mesenteric veins to the liver, where it is destroyed. The male *S. mansoni* is more susceptible to this killing effect than the female, but this will prevent the production of eggs at any rate.
Niridazole (Ambilhar)	Niridazole possesses both schistosomicidal and amebicidal properties. In addition, it has antiinflammatory properties and is a potent inhibitor of cell-mediated responses. It destroys the vitellogenic gland and egg production in the female and spermatogenesis in the male. It is highly effective against *Schistosoma haematobium*. Niridazole is extensively metabolized in the liver, and numerous toxicities do occur, especially in patients with impaired liver function. It causes hemolytic anemia in patients with glucose-6-phosphate dehydrogenase deficiency. It should be used cautiously in diseases involving the CNS, such as epilepsy.

▪ Table 37-2 ▪ Pharmacologic Properties of Antimalarial Agents

Antimalarial Drugs	Properties
Chloroquine (Arlen), amodiaquine (Camoquin), as an alternate drug	Chloroquine destroys schizonts in erythrocytes by interfering with DNA synthesis. The phosphate salts are active orally, whereas the hydrochloride salt is used for IV purposes. It accumulates in normal and parasitized erythrocytes. Overdosage has caused reversible corneal damage and permanent retinal damage. In toxic doses, chloroquine causes visual disturbances, hyperexcitability, convulsions, and heart block. It is an antimalarial of choice in all cases except chloroquine-resistant *Plasmodium falciparum*. In addition, it has a certain degree of effectiveness in amebiasis and in the late stages of rheumatoid arthritis.
Primaquine	Primaquine attacks plasmodia in the exoerthrocytic stages. It is effective for preventing relapse and as a prophylactic measure when staying in an infested area. Primaquine may cause hemolytic anemia, especially in patients who are deficient in glucose-6-phosphate dehydrogenase.
Quinine	Quinine is a naturally occurring alkaloid obtained from *Cinchona* bark, with a mechanism of action similar to that of chloroquine. Quinine is very useful in treating chloroquinine-resistant *Plasmodium falciparum*. In toxic doses, it may cause cinchonism characterized by tinnitus, headache, nausea, and visual disturbances.
Pyrimethamine (Daraprim)	Pyrimethamine is a folic acid antagonist with pharmacologic actions similar to chloguanide, methotrexate, and trimethoprim. Pyrimethamine may be used in combination with sulfadoxine for suppression and with sulfadizine for treatment of chloroquine-resistant *Plasmodium falciparum*.

▪ Table 37-3 ▪ Select Pharmacologic Properties of Drugs Most Often Used in Tuberculosis

Drugs	Properties
Isoniazid	Isoniazid is bactericidal for growing tubercle bacilli, is absorbed orally, and is metabolized by acetylation. It is a structural analogue of pyridoxine and may cause pyridoxine deficiency, peripheral neuritis, and, in toxic doses, pyridoxine-responsive convulsions.
Streptomycin	Streptomycin is given intramuscularly. It exerts its effects only on extracellular tubercle bacilli. When combined with other drugs, it delays the emergence of streptomycin-resistant mutants. It is ototoxic and may cause deafness.
Rifampin	Rifampin is absorbed from the GI tract and is excreted mainly into bile. It binds to DNA-dependent RNA polymerase and inhibits RNA synthesis. In higher-than-therapeutic doses, rifampin may cause a flulike syndrome and thrombocytopenia.
Ethambutol	Ethambutol suppresses the growth of isoniazid- and streptomycin-resistant tubercle bacilli. The most important but not common side effects are optic neuritis, decreased visual acuity, and inability to perceive the color green.

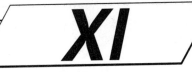

XI

Antiviral Agents, Immunopharmacology, and Cancer Chemotherapy

CHAPTER 38

Antiviral Agents

The antiviral agents consist of the following:

- Zidovudine (azidothymidine) (AZT)
- Acyclovir
- Ganciclovir
- Vidarbine (adenine arabinoside) (arz A)
- Idoxuridine
- Trifluridine
- Amantadine
- Rimantadine
- Ribavirin

Zidovudine

Zidovudine (Retrovir) is active against **human immunodeficiency virus type I** and other **retroviruses.** The drug inhibits the Epstein-Barr virus but not the herpes simplex or varicella-zoster virus. Zidovudine is phosphorylated to deoxynucleoside triphosphate, and hence inhibits the viral RNA-dependent DNA polymerase (**reverse transcriptase**). Zidovudine use can lead to granulocytopenia and anemia. Delayed neurotoxic reactions (seizures and Wernicke's encephalopathy) have been reported in connection with its use.

Acyclovir Sodium

Acyclovir inhibits viral replication by inhibiting DNA synthesis. It interacts with the virus-induced enzyme, especially **thymidine kinase** and **DNA polymerase.**

Acyclovir is effective in the treatment of herpes simplex virus type 1 and type 2 infections, including chronic and recurrent mucocutaneous herpes and in the immunologically impaired host, primary, and secondary genital herpes, neonatal herpes, and herpes simplex encephalitis.

Idoxuridine

Idoxuridine (Herplex and Stoxil) resembles thymidine in that its phosphorylated derivatives are incorporated into the viral DNA. Idoxuridine is effective against primarily the herpesviruses and poxviruses. It is administered topically in the treatment of herpes simplex keratitis but is too toxic to be given systematically, since it will precipitate bone marrow depression and other serious complications.

Amantadine Hydrochloride

The antiviral activity of amantadine (Symmetrel) is restricted to the RNA viruses, especially influenza type A. It exerts its effects by preventing the penetration and uncoating of the virus. ■ **Fig. 38-1** ■ Amantadine may be used either prophylactically or therapeutically in influenza type A virus. It is absorbed well from the GI tract and is eliminated extensively (90%) by the kidneys. The doses of amantadine should be reduced in patients with renal failure. Amantadine, which releases catecholamine, may cause insomnia, nervousness, dizziness, and ataxia when taken in toxic doses.

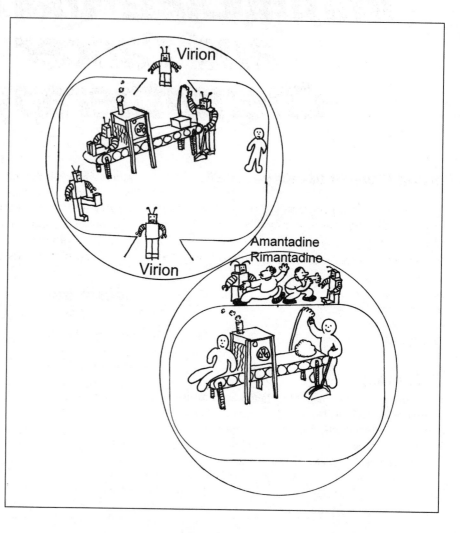

■ Fig. 38-1 ■
Amantadine prevents the
duplication of virus.

Immunopharmacology and Cancer Chemotherapy

Immunopharmacology

The immune system protects the body from bacteria, viruses, and other harmful microorganisms. It is also able to attack a healthy body and cause life-threatening diseases such as **multiple sclerosis.**

■ **Fig. 39-1** ■ In the past, immunosuppressive agents were used solely in patients undergoing **allotransplantation.** However, a new understanding of the role of **interleukins** in the pathophysiology of diseases has spawned new applications for these agents. Moreover, because tissue transplantation, including

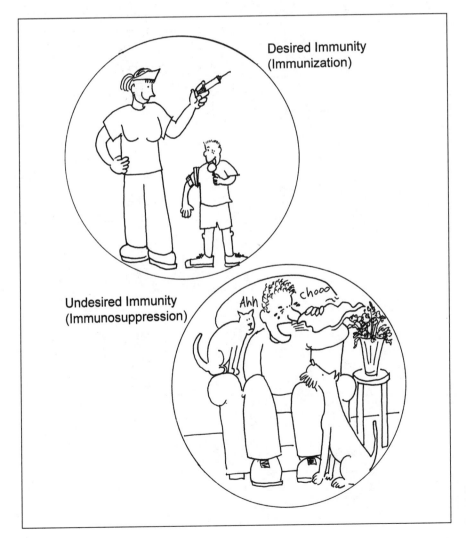

Desired Immunity
(Immunization)

Undesired Immunity
(Immunosuppression)

■ **Fig. 39-1** ■
Immunologic means of
disease control.

even bone marrow transplantation, is associated with complications and because the pharmacokinetics of agents are modified in organ transplant patients, an even greater understanding of the therapeutic refinements of immunomodulating agents is required.

Radioimmunotherapy

Radioimmunotherapy or monoclonal antibody-mediated radioimmunotherapy is a process that couples an antibody to a radioactive isotope in order to enhance its tumoricidal activity. The long-range beta emitters **rhenium 90Y and 188** have replaced iodine 131 as isotopes.

Cell Transfer Therapy and Cancer

Cell transfer therapy is a new approach to strengthening the innate ability of the immune system to fight against cancer. ■ **Fig. 39-2** ■ In this therapy, lymphocytes are isolated and cultured with interleukin-2 for 3 days to yield lymphokine-activated killer cells, which are then administered to patients along with interleukin-2.

Immunosuppressive Agents

The following agents and measures are used for immunosuppressive therapy: corticosteroids, cytotoxic agents (alkylating agents and antimetabolites), cyclosporin A and dihydrocyclosporin C, antilymphocyte globulin and Rho (D) immune globulin (RhoGAM), lymphoid irradiation and thoracic duct drainage, and immunomodulating agents (interferons and their inducers). ■ **Fig. 39-3** ■

Immunosuppressive agents are used in patients undergoing **organ transplantation,** such as of the liver, heart, and kidney. One or a combination of agents may be given, including **glucocorticosteroids, azathioprine,** and **cyclophosphamide.** In addition, a combination of drug therapy and other ameliorative techniques that bring about lymphocyte depletion, such as thoracic duct drainage or total lymph node irradiation, may be indicated.

Immunosuppressive agents are used in the treatment of **autoimmune diseases.** For example, the treatment

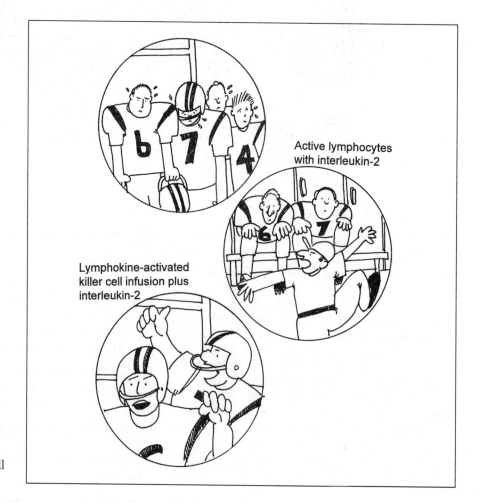

Active lymphocytes with interleukin-2

Lymphokine-activated killer cell infusion plus interleukin-2

■ **Fig. 39-2** ■
Use of lymphokine in cell transfer therapy.

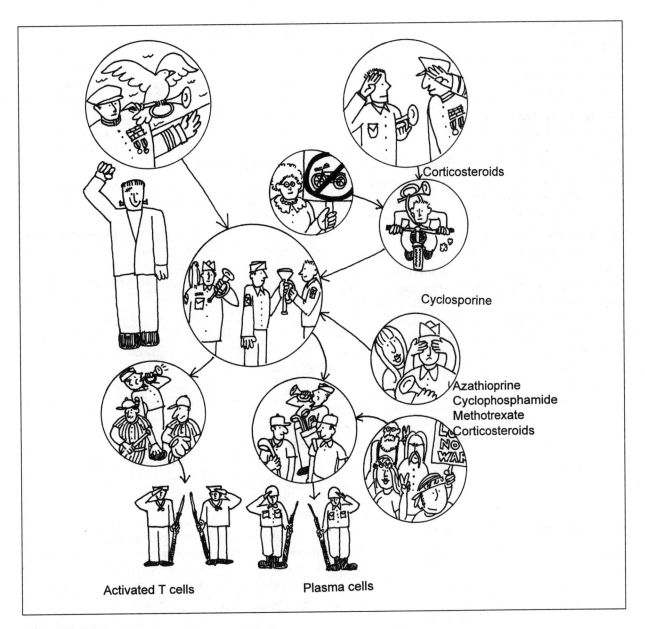

Activated T cells   Plasma cells

■ **Fig. 39-3** ■

Sites of action of immunosuppressive agents.

approach to **chronic active hepatitis** not attributable to drugs, **Wilson's disease,** or alpha$_1$-antitrypsin deficiency consists of prednisone combined with azathioprine. Azathioprine by itself is not effective in this disorder. **Idiopathic thrombocytopenic purpura** is treated with corticosteroids and splenectomy, and immunosuppressive agents are used in refractory cases. **Hemolysis** due to warm-reacting autoimmune antibodies (autoimmune hemolytic anemia) involving immunoglobulin G (predominantly IgG$_1$ and IgG$_3$) is initially treated with prednisone. If this proves

unsuccessful, splenectomy (in younger patients) or immunosuppression using azathioprine or cyclophosphamide (in older patients) is next carried out.

The Corticosteroids

Corticosteroids have the following pharmacologic effects on immunosuppression:

■ They inhibit prostaglandin E$_2$ and leukotriene synthesis.

■ They reduce the macrophage-mediated lysosomal contents.

- They reduce the activity of the lymphocyte-mediated chemotactic factor and lymphotoxin.
- They increase the catabolism of immunoglobulin such as IgG.
- They are able to lyse T-helper cells.
- They interfere with the ability of reticuloendothelial macrophages to attack and destroy antibody-coated cells.

The Cytotoxic Compounds

Alkylating Agents - Cyclophosphamide (Cytoxan) and its active metabolites destroy the rapidly proliferating lymphocytes and hence are potent immunosuppressive agents.

Antimetabolites - When injected, **azathioprine** (Imuran) is rapidly converted to **6-mercaptopurine.** The half-life of azathioprine after IV injection is 10–20 minutes, and that of 6-mercaptopurine is somewhat longer. The **cytotoxic activity** of these thiopurines is due to the conversion of mercaptopurine to 6-thiouric acid, a noncarcinostatic metabolite. Azathioprine depresses bone marrow functioning, its chief side effect.

Cyclosporin A - Cyclosporin A has been used as the sole immunosuppressant (without prednisone or other drugs) for cadaveric transplants of the kidney, pancreas, and liver. Cyclosporin A has been observed to cause reversible hepatic toxicity and nephrotoxicity.

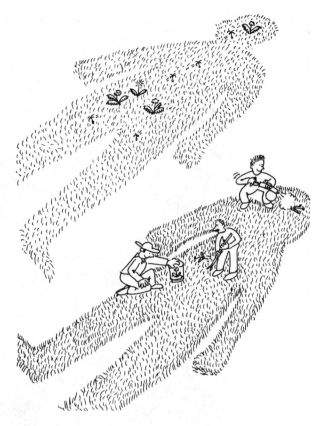

■ **Fig. 39-4** ■
Antineoplastic agents suppressing the growth and spread of malignant cells.

Cancer and Its Treatment

Approaches to Cancer Therapy

Malignant neoplastic diseases may be treated by various approaches: surgery, radiation therapy, immunotherapy, or chemotherapy, or a combination of these. The extent of a malignant disease (staging) should be ascertained in order to plan an effective therapeutic intervention. ■ **Fig. 39-4** ■

Chemotherapy

Cytotoxic drugs are not specific in their actions. Not only do they arrest cancerous cells, but they also arrest normal cells, especially those of the rapidly proliferating tissues, such as the bone marrow, lymphoid system, oral and GI epithelium, skin and hair follicles, and germinal epithelia of the gonads. Consequently, the therapeutic regimen must be carried out using **high-dose intermittent schedules,** not a low-dose continuous approach. Succeeding doses are given as soon as the patient has recovered from the previous treatment.

Antineoplastic agents may be **teratogenic, carcinogenic,** or **immunosuppressant,** and they exert their lethal effects on different phases of cell cycle by being either **cell-cycle specific** or **nonspecific.** ■ **Fig. 39-5** ■

Alkylating Agents

The alkylating agents exert their antineoplastic actions by generating highly reactive carbonium ion intermediates that form a covalent linkage with various nucleophilic components on both proteins and DNA. The 7 position of the purine base **guanine** is particularly susceptible to alkylation, resulting in miscoding, depurination, or ring cleavage.

Nitrogen Mustards - The activity of nitrogen mustards depends on the presence of a bis-(2-chloroethyl) grouping, present in **mechlorethamine** (Mustargen), which is used in patients with Hodgkin's disease and other lymphomas, usually in combination with other drugs, such as in **MOPP therapy** (mechlorethamine, Oncovin [vincristine], procarbazine, and predinose). It may cause bone marrow depression.

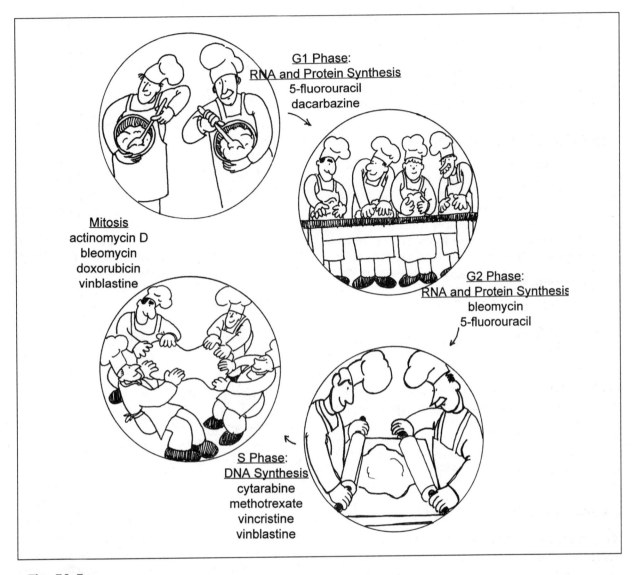

■ Fig. 39-5 ■
Actions of antineoplastic agents on the cell cycle.

Chlorambucil - Chlorambucil (Leukeran), the least toxic nitrogen mustard, is used as the drug of choice in the treatment of chronic lymphocytic leukemia. It is absorbed orally, is slow in its onset of action, and may cause bone marrow depression.

Cyclophosphamide - Cyclophosphamide (Cytoxan and Endoxan) is used in the treatment of Hodgkin's disease, lymphosarcoma, and other lymphomas. It is employed as a secondary drug in patients with acute leukemia and in combination with doxorubicin in women with breast cancer. A drug combination effective in the treatment of breast cancer is cyclophosphamide, methotrexate, fluorouracil, and prednisone.

Alkyl Sulfonate - Because it produces selective myelosuppression, it is used in cases of chronic myelocytic leukemia.

Nitrosoureas - Carmustine (BCNU), lomustine (CCNU), and semustine are lipid soluble, cross the blood-brain barrier, and are therefore effective in treating brain tumors. They are bone marrow depressants.

Antimetabolites

Folic Acid Analogues - **Methotrexate** (Amethopterin) is a folic acid antagonist that binds to dihydrofolate reductase, thus interfering with the synthesis of the active cofactor tetrahydrofolic acid, which is necessary for the synthesis of thymidylate, purine nucleotides, and the amino acids serine and methionine.

The effects of methotrexate may be reversed by the administration of **leucovorin,** the reduced folate. This **leucovorin "rescue"** prevents or reduces the toxicity of methotrexate, which is expressed as mouth lesions (stomatitis), injury to the GI epithelium (diarrhea), leukopenia, and thrombocytopenia.

Pyrimidine Analogues - **Fluorouracil** and **fluorodeoxyuridine** (floxuridine) inhibit pyrimidine nucleotide biosynthesis and interfere with the synthesis and actions of nucleic acids. To exert its effect, fluorouracil (5-FU) must first be converted to nucleotide derivatives such as **5-fluorodeoxyuridylalte** (5-FdUMP).

Similarly, **floxuridine** (FUdR) is also converted to FdUMP by the following reactions:

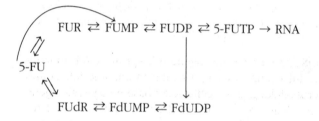

FdUMP inhibits **thymidylate synthetase,** and this in turn inhibits the essential formation of dTTP, one of the four precursors of DNA. In addition, 5-fluorouracil is sequentially converted to 5-FUTP, which becomes incorporated into RNA, thus inhibiting its processing and fuctioning.

Fluorouracil is used for the following types of cancer:

- Breast carcinoma
- Colon carcinoma
- Gastric adenocarcinoma
- Hepatocellular carcinoma
- Pancreatic adenocarcinoma

Because 5-fluorouracil is metabolized rapidly in the liver, it is administered intravenously and not orally. 5-fluorouracil causes myelosuppression and mucositis.

Deoxycytidine Analogues - Cytosine arabinoside (Cytarbine, Cytosar, and Ara-C) is an analogue of deoxycytidine, differing only in its substitution of sugar arabinose for deoxyribose. It is converted to Ara-CTP and thereby inhibits DNA-polymerase according to the following reactions:

$$\text{Ara-C} \xrightarrow{\text{Deoxycytidine kinase}} \text{Ara-CMP} \xrightarrow{\text{dCMP kinase}} \text{Ara-CDP}$$
$$\text{Ara-CDP} \xrightarrow{\text{NDP kinase}} \text{Ara-CTP}$$
$$\text{Deoxynucleotides} \xrightarrow[\text{DNA-polymerase}]{\text{//}} \text{DNA}$$

Cytosine arabinoside is used in the treatment of **acute granulocytic leukemia**. Doxorubicin; daunorubicin and cytarabine; cytarabine and thioguanine; or cytarabine, vincristine, and prednisone are the combinations of agents employed.

Resistance to cytosine arabinoside may stem from the following factors:

The deletion of deoxycytidine kinase
An increased intracellular pool of dCTP, a nucleotide that competes with Ara-CTP
Increased cytidine deaminase activity, converting Ara-C to inactive Ara-U

The toxic effects of cytosine arabinoside are myelosuppression and injury to the gastrointestinal epithelium, which causes nausea, vomiting, and diarrhea.

Purine Antimetabolites - 6-Mercaptopurine (6MP) and 6-thioguanine (6TG) are analogues of the purines, hypoxanthine and guanine, which must be activated by nucleotide formation, according to the following scheme:

$$\text{6-MP} + \text{phosphoribosylpyrophosphate (PRPP)} \xrightarrow{\substack{\text{Hypoxanthine - guanine} \\ \text{phosphoribosyl transferase}}}$$
$$\text{6 ThiolMP}$$

$$\text{6TG} + \text{PRPP} \longrightarrow \text{6 ThioGMP}$$

6-Mercaptopurine is used in the treatment of acute lymphoid leukemia. Its chief toxicities are hepatic damage and bone marrow depression.

Thioguanine is used in patients with acute granulocytic leukemia, usually in combination with cytosine arabinoside and daunorubicin.

Natural Products

Vinca Alkaloids - The vinca alkaloids (**vinblastine, vincristine,** and **vindesine**), which bind to tubulin, block mitosis with metaphase arrest. Vinca alkaloids are used for the following types of cancer:

Acute lymphoid leukemia: In the induction phase, vincristine is used with prednisone.
Acute myelomonocytic or monocytic leukemia: Cytarabine, vincristine, and prednisone.

Hodgkin's disease: Mechlorethamine, Oncovin (vincristine), procarbazine, and prednisone (MOPP).

Nodular lymphoma: Cyclophosphamide, Oncovin (vincristine), and prednisone (CVP).

Diffuse histiocytic lymphoma: Cyclophosphamide, Adriamycin (doxorubicin), vincristine, and prednisone (**CHOP**); bleomycin, Adriamycin (doxorubicin), cyclophosphamide, Oncovin (vincristine), and prednisone (**BACOP**); or cyclophosphamide, Oncovin (vincristine), methotrexate, and cytarabine (**COMA**).

Wilms' tumor: Dactinomycin and vincristine.

Ewing's sarcoma: Cyclophosphamide, dactinomycin, or vincristine.

Embryonal rhabdomyosarcoma: Cyclophosphamide, dactinomycin, or vincristine.

Bronchogenic carcinoma: Doxorubicin, cyclophosphamide, and vincristine.

The chief toxicity associated with vinblastine use is bone marrow depression. The toxicity of vincristine consists of paresthesia, neuritic pain, muscle weakness, and visual disturbances. In addition, both vinblastine and vincristine may cause alopecia.

Dactinomycin - The antibiotics that bind to DNA are nonspecific to the cell-cycle phase. Dactinomycin binds to double-stranded DNA and prevents RNA synthesis by inhibiting DNA-dependent RNA polymerase.

It is administered intravenously in the treatment for pediatric solid tumors such as Wilms' tumor and rhabdomyosarcoma and for gestational choriocarcinoma.

Mithramycin - The mechanism of action of mithramycin (Mithracin) is similar to dactinomycin's. It is used in patients with advanced disseminated tumors of the testis and for the treatment of hypercalcemia associated with cancer.

Daunorubicin and Doxorubicin - Daunorubicin (Daunomycin and Cerubidine) and doxorubicin (Adriamycin) bind to and cause the intercalation of the DNA molecule, thereby inhibiting DNA template function. They also provoke DNA chain scission and chromosomal damage.

Daunorubicin is useful in treating patients with acute lymphocytic or acute granulocytic leukemia. Adriamycin is useful in cases of solid tumors such as sarcoma, metastatic breast cancer, and thyroid cancer. These agents cause stomatitis, alopecia, myelosuppression, and cardiac abnormalities ranging from arrythmias to cardiomyopathy.

Cis-Platinum - Cis-platinum (cisplatin) binds to intracellular DNA, causing both interstrand and intrastrand cross-linking. It is a cell-cycle phase nonspecific agent. Cis-platinum, which is ineffective orally, is used for testicular, bladder, and head and neck cancers. It precipitates nephrotoxicity, ototoxicity, and GI injury.

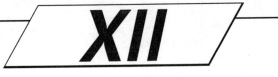

XII

Poisons and Antidotes

CHAPTER 40

Treatment of Poisoning

Agricultural Poisons

Polycyclic Chlorinated Insecticides

The polycyclic chlorinated insecticides include chlordane, heptachlor, dieldrin, and aldrin. The clinical manifestations of toxicity include hyperexcitability, ataxia, tremors, and convulsions. Treatment includes emesis and the administration of activated charcoal followed by gastric lavage along with anticonvulsants (**diazepam**).

Cholinesterase Inhibitors Used as Insecticides

The cholinesterase inhibitors are divided into two categories: **organophosphorus compounds,** such as parathion, malathion, and tetraethyl pyrophosphate (TEPP), and the **carbamates,** such as naphthyl-*N*-methyl carbamate (carbaryl and Sevin).

The clinical manifestations of acute and severe poisoning from the organophosphorus insecticides include **cholinergic crisis,** resulting from the stimulation of muscarinic cholinergic receptors (bronchoconstriction, salivation, sweating, lacrimation, bradycardia, hypotension, and urinary and fecal incontinence), from the stimulation of nicotinic cholinergic receptors (muscular fasciculation), and from CNS effects (with initial restlessness, tremors, ataxia, and convulsions, followed by CNS depression and respiratory and circulatory depression). The treatment of a cholinergic crisis caused by organophosphorus compounds includes the administration of a cholinesterase reactivator such as pralidoxine (2-PAM) together with atropine. See ■ **Fig. 4-6** ■ The poisoning stemming from antidoting with 2-PAM can be avoided in the event of carbaryl toxicity, because this agent is a reversible cholinesterase inhibitor (see Chap. 4).

Herbicides

The herbicides include **paraquat** (Methyl Viologen) and diquat and are inactivated by contact with soil. Paraquat may be absorbed transdermally. The ingestion of paraquat causes GI upset, respiratory distress, hemoptysis, ulceration of the pharynx, and cyanosis. Besides causing GI and pulmonary distress as well as cardiac arrhythmias, diquat may also precipitate oliguria and progressive renal failure. The treatment of toxicity, which must be initiated early, includes the administration of activated charcoal followed by lavage with a 1% **bentonite solution,** the administration of **hydrocortisone** and **furosemide,** and hemodialysis.

Industrial Poisons: Alcohols and Glycol

Ethyl Alcohol

Ethyl alcohol is mostly metabolized by alcohol dehydrogenase and exhibits zero-order kinetics (10 mg/hour). There is no known antidote. **Disulfiram** (Antabuse) inhibits **aldehyde dehydrogenase** and should never be used in combination with ethyl alcohol.

Methyl Alcohol

Methyl alcohol is mostly metabolized by alcohol dehydrogenase to formaldehyde and formic acid, and poisoning causes blindness and acidosis. Ethyl alcohol, when given IV, competes with methyl alcohol, and promotes its excretion unchanged by the kidneys.

Ethylene Glycol

Ethylene glycol causes an inebriation resembling that of ethyl alcohol and is followed by vomiting, cyanosis, hypotension, tachycardias, tachypnea, pulmonary edema, acidosis, anuria (calcium oxalate crystals), convulsions, and unconsciousness. Death results from respiratory failure or irreversible brain damage, or both. Ethyl alcohol may be used as an antidote to ethylene glycol poisoning. After this life-supporting step has been taken, additional supportive treatment consists of treating the acidosis, pulmonary edema, anuria, and hypoglycemia.

Isopropyl Alcohol

The symptoms of isopropyl alcohol poisoning are similar to those for ethyl alcohol, but there is a more marked depression of the CNS. Other symptoms include persistent nausea, vomiting, hematemesis, abdominal pain, dehydration, depression respiration, and oliguria. Emergency treatment includes artificial respiration and hemodialysis. Additional supportive therapy includes correcting the electrolyte imbalance, maintaining blood pressure, correcting the oliguria, and preventing renal failure.

The Halogenated Hydrocarbons

Carbon Tetrachloride - Carbon tetrachloride decomposes to **phosgene** and hydrochloric acid. In general, carbon tetrachloride inflicts injury on all organs, especially the **kidneys** (marked edema and fatty degeneration of the tubules) and the **liver** (centrilobular necrosis and fatty degeneration). The toxic manifestations include oliguria, jaundice, and coma. Carbon tetrachloride oliguria is followed by a prolonged period of diuresis. The complete restoration of hepatic and renal functions is possible but takes place slowly. The treatment of poisoning consists of basic supportive treatment. Sympathomimetic agents should not be given for the hypotension, as cardiac arrhythmia may ensue.

Trichloroethylene - Trichloroethylene causes CNS depression and unconsciousness. Respiration and circulation should be supported in affected patients, but recovery is prompt without leaving residual injuries.

Petroleum and Solvent Distillates - The excessive inhalation or ingestion of petroleum products causes nausea, vomiting, and pulmonary irritation (coughing, hemoptysis, and CNS and respiratory depression). Treatment of the poisoning includes the early administration of activated charcoal and gastric lavage, artificial respiration, and any other therapy that will minimize pulmonary injury.

Aromatic Hydrocarbons

The aromatic hydrocarbons include **benzene, xylene,** and **toluene.** Prolonged exposure to benzene and toluene causes anemia. The ingestion of these agents provokes GI symptoms, dizziness, headache, ataxia, delirium, cardiac irregularities, paralysis, and convulsions. The treatment of toxicity includes administering **diazepam** to control the convulsions, providing supportive therapy, and monitoring the hematopoietic elements.

Corrosives

The corrosives include both acidic and basic substances such as **chlorine** and **hydrochloric acid.** The clinical manifestations of corrosive poisoning include burning pain in the mouth, pharynx, and abdomen; severe hypotension; asphyxia; perforation of the esophagus or stomach; peritonitis; and, once the patient is recovered, strictures of the esophagus or stomach. Treatment of corrosive toxicity consists of diluting it with water or milk. Gastric lavage, emesis, and the use of **chemical antidotes** (acid for base and base for acid) will compound injury and are **absolutely contraindicated.** The circulation should be sustained by the transfusion of 5% glucose in saline, and nutrition should be supplied by IV administration of carbohydrates.

Metal Poisoning

Lead Toxicity

The treatment of toxicity includes the administration of **calcium disodium edetate** (Calcium Disodium Versensate) and **D-penicillamine** (Cuprimine). Although D-penicillamine is not as active as dimercaprol, it is more active when given orally and hence is useful for the long-term deleading of patients over the course of several months.

Mercury Toxicity

The treatment of choice includes **dimercaprol** (BAL) or **D-penicillamine** (Cuprimine), or both.

Arsenic Toxicity

The recommended treatment includes dimercaprol.

Treatment of Heavy Metal Poisoning

Chelating Agents - Among the heavy metal chelators, the following have been used extensively. **Penicillamine** chelates copper, mercury, lead, and iron. It is effective for the removal of copper in patients with Wilson's disease. **Deferoxamine** chelates iron. Dimercaptrol is effective in the treatment of poisoning due to mercury, arsenic, or gold. It should not be used in poisoning caused by cadmium, iron, or selenium. Dimercaprol is metabolized in the liver, but high concentrations inhibit cellular respiration.

Calcium Disodium EDTA - Calcium disodium EDTA is not metabolized and not active orally. EDTA penetrates cell membranes relatively poorly and therefore chelates extracellular metal ions much more effectively than intracellular ions. It is therefore administered by IV drip. Adverse reactions to EDTA include renal damage, hypersensitivity, and transient bone marrow depression.

The Asphyxiants

Carbon Monoxide

The affinity of hemoglobin for carbon monoxide is 200 times greater than that for oxygen. At approximately a 60% saturation of hemoglobin with carbon monoxide, convulsions, coma, and respiratory failure arise. Treatment includes administering 100% oxygen in conjunction with artificial respiration for 1–2 hours and maintaining the patient's body temperature and blood pressure. The **cerebral edema** that may occur should be treated with **mannitol** and **prednisone.** The convulsions may be effectively controlled with **diazepam.**

Cyanide

The treatment of cyanide poisoning includes the production of methemoglobin, which can then compete with cytochrome oxidase for the cyanide ions. This goal may be achieved through the IV administration of **sodium nitrite** or, if this is not available, with any nitrite, given by inhalation. The cyanide should be detoxified by causing it to react with **thiosulfate** to form the much less toxic **thiocyanate.**

Index

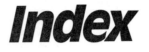

Numbers followed by the letter *f* indicate figures; numbers followed by the letter *t* indicate tables.

Abbokinase, 105
Abdominal distention, treatment of, 19
Abortifacients, 150
Abscess, treatment of, 166
Absence seizures, treatment of, 42–44
Accelerated growth, androgens to treat, 132
Acebutolol
  antiarrhythmic effects of, 92, 93, 93t
  characteristics of, 28t
Acenocoumarol, 103
Acetazolamide, 95
  site of action of, 97t
Acetphenolisatin, laxative effects of, 139
Acetylcholine, 17, 19f
  actions of, 32
  drug interactions of, 7
  receptors for, 17–18
Acetylcholinesterase, 17
Acetylcysteine, mucolytic effects of, 144
Achlorhydria, 5
  B_{12} deficiency from, 107
Acid pepsin disease, 137
Acidosis, reversal of, 115
Acne, estrogens to treat, 131
Actinomycosis, treatment of, 163
Activated charcoal, to treat poisoning, 183, 184
Acute granulocytic leukemia, treatment of, 179
Acute lymphoid leukemia, treatment of, 178, 179
Acute myelomonocytic leukemia, treatment of, 178
Acyclovir, antiviral effects of, 171
Adapin, 56
Adenine arabinoside, antiviral effects of, 171
Adenosine, functions of, 147
Adenylate cyclase, 151
Adrenal steroids
  classification of, 116–117
  contraindications to, 120
  indications for, 117–120, 119f
  mechanism of action of, 117–120, 121f
  side effects of, 120f
Adrenergic neuron blockers, antihypertensive effects of, 98, 99
Adrenergic receptors
  agonists of, 27–28
  antagonists of, 28
  types of, 27
Adrenergic transmission, 25–28
  blocking of, 28
Adrenocorticotropic hormone (ACTH), 152
Adriamycin, 178, 179
Agar, laxative effects of, 139
Agonist, defined, 6
AIDS, treatment of, 171
Akathisia, 49
Albumin, drug binding by, 5, 13
Albuterol, to treat asthma, 141

Alcohol
  cardiovascular effects of, 84
  central nervous system effects of, 83–84
  GI effects of, 84
  liver effects of, 85
  pharmacokinetics of, 85
  toxicity of, 183, 184
Alcohol withdrawal, treatment of, 54
Alcoholism, treatment of, 57
Aldactone, 96
  site of action of, 97t
Aldomet, 99
Aldosterone, 95, 116, 117
Aldosteronism
  primary, 117f
  secondary, 118f
Aldrin, poisoning by, 183
Alendonate sodium, to treat osteoporosis, 127
Alkyl sulfonate, 177
Alkylating agents
  cytotoxic effects of, 176
  immunosuppressive effects of, 174
  pharmacology of, 176–177
Allergic reactions, 12
Allergies, treatment of, 28
Allopurinol
  indications for, 73
  to treat gout, 10
Alopecia, treatment of, 99
Alpha methyldopa, 26
  antihypertensive effects of, 98, 99
Alpha-adrenergic blockers, 28
  antihypertensive effects of, 98
Alpha-methyldopamine, 27
Alpha-methylhistamine, 147
Alpha-methylnorepinephrine, 27
Alpha-methyltyrosine, 25
Alprazolam, 59
Amantadine, 33, 36
  antiviral effects of, 171, 172f
  to treat neuroleptic malignant syndrome, 52
Ambilhar, 167t
Amenorrhea
  hypothalamic, 129
  treatment of, 131, 132
Amethopterin, 177
Amiloride, 95, 96
  site of action of, 97t
Aminoglycosides
  mechanism of action of, 157
  pharmacology of, 163
Aminophylline, to treat asthma, 141, 152
Amiodarone, antiarrhythmic effects of, 92, 93t, 94
Amitriptyline, 56
Amlodipine, calcium-blocking effect of, 153

Ammonium carbonate, expectorant effects of, 144
Ammonium chloride, expectorant effects of, 144
Amobarbital, sedative effects of, 85
Amodiaquine, to treat malaria, 168t
Amoeba infection, treatment of, 164
Amoebic dysentery, treatment of, 166
Amoebic hepatitis, treatment of, 166
Amoxapine, 59
Amoxicillin, 162
    side effects of, 163
    to treat ulcer, 138
Amphetamines
    excretion of, 9
    as sympathomimetic, 28
Amphotericin B
    indications for, 166
    mechanism of action of, 157
    pharmacology of, 165
Ampicillin, 162
    side effects of, 163
Amrinone, to treat congestive heart failure, 91
Anabolism, androgens to regulate, 132
Analgesics, 71–74
    blood-brain barrier and, 6
    narcotic, 67–70
Ancobon, 165
Androgen-binding protein, synthesis of, 129
Androgens, 132
    antagonists of, 133
    side effects of, 133
Anectine, muscle relaxant effects of, 79
Anemia, 106
    treatment of, 106–107
Anesthetic(s), 74–77
    blood-brain barrier and, 6
    epinephrine as, 28
    general, 74–75
    local, 76–77
    spinal, 76, 77f
Angina pectoris, treatment of, 101–102, 154
Angiotensin II, 11
Angiotensin-converting enzyme inhibitors, 98, 100f
Anipamil, calcium-blocking effect of, 153
Anise oil, expectorant effects of, 144
Anisindione, 103
Antabuse, 183
Antacids, 137
    drug interactions of, 12
Antagonist, defined, 6
Antepar, 167t
Anthrax, treatment of, 163
Antiarrhythmics, 92–94
    drug interactions of, 154
Antiasthmatics, 141–143, 152
Antibiotics
    drug interactions of, 158
    mechanisms of action of, 157
    spectra of activity of, 158
    types of, 159–164
Anticholinergics, 19–21
    contraindications to, 24–25
    side effects of, 25f
    to treat asthma, 141
    to treat parkinsonism, 36
    to treat ulcer, 137
Anticoagulants, 103
    contraindications to, 104
    indications for, 104–105
Antidepressants, 56–63
    MAO inhibitors, 58–59

new types of, 58–59
    tricyclic, 56–58
Antidiuretic hormone (ADH), 95, 130, 152
Antiemetics, 138–139
Antiestrogens, 131–132
Antifertility agents, 132
Antifungals, 165
Antihelminthics, 167t
Antihistamines, drug interactions of, 12
Antihypertensives
    classes of, 98
    pharmacology of, 98–100
Antiinflammatories, 71–74
Antilymphocyte globulin, immunosuppressive effects of, 174
Antimalarials, 168t
Antimetabolites
    cytotoxic effects of, 176
    immunosuppressive effects of, 174
    mechanism of action of, 157
    pharmacology of, 177–178
Antimicrobial therapy, 157–164
Antiminth, 167t
Antimonials, pentavalent, indications for, 166
Antineoplastic agents
    actions of, 177f
    types of, 176
Antipyretics, 71–74
    to treat thyrotoxic crisis, 124
Antitussives, 70, 144
Anturane, indications for, 73
Anxiety, treatment of, 53–54, 54f
Anxiolytics, 53–55
Apresoline, 99
Ara-A, antiviral effects of, 171
Ara-C, 178
Arachidonic acid, 149
Aralen, to treat malaria, 168t
L-aromatic amino acid decarboxylase, 25
Aromatic diamidines, indications for, 166
Aromatic hydrocarbons, poisoning by, 184
Arrhythmia, treatment of, 92–94
Arsenic, poisoning by, 184
Artane
    anticholinergic effects of, 50
    to treat parkinsonism, 36
Arteriolar vasodilators, antihypertensive effects of, 98, 99
Artificial valves, anticoagulant use with, 104
Ascariasis, treatment of, 167t
Ascorbic acid. See Vitamin C
Asphyxiants, poisoning by, 185
Aspirin
    anticoagulant effect of, 150
    drug interactions of, 14
    effects of, 71
    indications for, 71, 73
    side effects of, 72–73
    transport of, 5
Astemizole, histamine₁ receptor drug, 147
Asthma
    cAMP and, 152
    treatment of, 141–143, 152
Atenolol, antiadrenergic activity of, 27t, 28t
Athrombin-K, 103
Atrial fibrillation, treatment of, 104
Atrial natriuretic factor (ANF), 95
Atromid S, anticholesterol effects of, 108
Atrophic vaginitis, estrogens to treat, 131
Atropine
    anticholinergic effects of, 19, 21
    dose-dependent effects of, 22–23

drug interactions of, 7
  toxicity of, 23
    to treat diarrhea, 140
    to treat digitalis toxicity, 90
Auranofin, indications for, 73
Aurothioglucose, indications for, 73
Autacoids, 147–148
Autoimmune diseases, treatment of, 174
Autonomic nervous system, 17
  drugs affecting, 17–28
Aventyl, 56
Axid, to treat ulcer, 137
Azathioprine
  cytotoxic effects of, 176
  immunosuppressive effects of, 174, 175
Azelastine, histamine$_1$ receptor blocking drug, 147
Azidothymidine (AZT), antiviral effects of, 171
Azlocillin, 162
Azodipine, calcium-blocking effect of, 153

Bacitracin
  drug interactions of, 158
  mechanism of action of, 157
Baclofen, muscle relaxant effects of, 79
BACOP regimen, indications for, 178
Bacteremia, treatment of, 163
Bacteroides infection, treatment of, 163, 164
Bacteroides fragilis infection, treatment of, 162
BAL, to treat poisoning, 184
Barbiturates
  anesthetic effect of, 74
  effects on bone, 127
  pharmacology of, 85
  safety of, 7, 8
  to treat epilepsy, 39–41
Batanopride, 139, 148
BCNU, 177
Beclomethasone, to treat asthma, 142, 143
Benadryl
  histamine$_1$ receptor drug, 147
  to treat dystonia, 50
Benemid, indications for, 73
Bentonite, to treat poisoning, 183
Benzene, poisoning by, 184
Benzimidazole derivatives, to treat ulcer, 137
Benzodiazepines
  anesthetic effect of, 74
  indications for, 44, 53–54, 55f
  mode of action of, 53
  side effects of, 55
Benzothiazepines, calcium-blocking effect of, 153
Benztropine, 24
  anticholinergic effects of, 50
  to treat parkinsonism, 36
Benzylpenicillin, 162
Beta-adrenergic blockers, 28
  antianginal effects of, 102
  antiarrhythmic effects of, 93–94
  antihypertensive effects of, 98
  to treat thyrotoxic crisis, 124
Beta-adrenergic receptor kinase (BARK), 151
Beta-arrestin, 151
Beta$_2$ stimulants, to treat asthma, 141, 152
Bethanechol, 18, 19
Bicarbonate, drug interactions of, 12, 14
Bilarcil, 167t
Biltricide, 167t
Bismuth subsalicylate, to treat diarrhea, 140
Bitolterol, to treat asthma, 141
Bladder cancer, treatment of, 179

Blastomyces infection, treatment of, 165
Bleomycin, indications for, 178, 179
Blood
  prostaglandin effects on, 149
  steroid effects on, 119
Blood flow, and drug absorption, 5
Blood pressure, control of, 98
Blood-brain barrier, 5, 6
Bone marrow transplantation, 174
Bordetella pertussis, toxin produced by, 151
Botulinum toxin, 17, 20f
Bradykinin, 148
Bran, laxative effects of, 139
Breast cancer, treatment of, 131, 132, 178, 179
Bretylium, antiarrhythmic effects of, 92, 93t, 94
Bromocriptine
  to treat neuroleptic malignant syndrome, 52
  to treat parkinsonism, 33, 35, 36f
Bronchial asthma, 141
  cAMP and, 152
Bronchodilators, to treat asthma, 141
Bronchogenic carcinoma, treatment of, 179
Brucellosis, treatment of, 164
Budenisone, to treat asthma, 143
Bumetanide, 95
Bupivacaine, anesthetic effect of, 76, 77
Bupropion, 59
Butoxamine, antiadrenergic activity of, 27t, 28t
Butyrylcholinesterase, 17

Caffeine, calcium-facilitating effect of, 153
Calcitonin, 122, 127, 152
Calcium
  agonists of, 153
  blockers of, 153, 154
  effects of, 152
  function of, 127
  and neurotransmitter release, 153
  serum levels of, 126t
  to treat osteoporosis, 127
Calcium channel(s), 153
Calcium channel blockers
  antianginal effects of, 101–102
  antihypertensive effects of, 98, 100, 100t
Calcium chloride, to treat hypoparathyroidism, 127
Calcium disodium edetate, to treat poisoning, 184–185
Calcium gluconate
  to treat hypocalcemia, 128f
  to treat hypoparathyroidism, 127
Calcium metabolism, steroid effects on, 120
Calmodulin, 152
Camoquin, to treat malaria, 168t
cAMP cascade, 151
Cancer
  cell transfer therapy for, 174
  chemotherapy for, 176–178
  treatment of, 10, 11, 176
Candida infection, treatment of, 165
Capillariasis, treatment of, 167t
Captopril
  antihypertensive effects of, 98, 100f
  endocrine effects of, 11
Carbachol, 18, 19
Carbamates, poisoning by, 183
Carbamazepine
  drug interactions of, 154
  to treat epilepsy, 40–41, 43f
Carbaryl, poisoning by, 183

Carbenicillin, 162
  indications for, 163
  side effects of, 163
Carbidopa, 25
  to treat neuroleptic malignant syndrome, 52
  to treat parkinsonism, 31, 32, 35
Carbimazole, to treat hyperthyroidism, 123
Carbon monoxide, poisoning by, 185
Carbon tetrachloride, poisoning by, 184
Carboprost, 150
Carboxymethylcellulose, laxative effects of, 139
Cardiac glycosides
  modes of action of, 89
  safety of, 7
  side effects of, 8, 90
Carmustine, 177
Carrier-mediated transport, 3
Cascara sagrada, laxative effects of, 139
Castor oil, laxative effects of, 139
Catapres, 100
Catechol-O-methyltransferase, 27
Catecholamines, 25
  metabolism of, 27
Cathartics, 139–140
CCNU, 177
Cefaclor, 163
Cefadroxil, 163
Cefamandole, 163
Cefazolin, 163
Cefotaxime, 163
Cefoxitin, 163
Cell transfer therapy, 174
Celontin, to treat seizures, 42
Central nervous system, 17
Cephalexin, 163
Cephaloridine, 163
Cephalosporin
  mechanism of action of, 157
  pharmacology of, 163
Cephalothin, 163
Cephaprin, 163
Cephradine, 163
Cerebral edema, treatment of, 185
Cerebral palsy, treatment of, 54
Cerubidine, 178
Cervical cancer, contraceptives and, 132
Cestode infection, treatment of, 167t
Cetirizine, histamine$_1$ receptor blocking drug, 147
Chagas' disease, treatment of, 166
Chancroid, treatment of, 164
Chemotherapy
  agents of, 10, 176–178
  mechanisms of, 157
Chlamydia infection, treatment of, 164
Chlorambucil, 177
Chloramphenicol
  drug interactions of, 158
  indications for, 163
  mechanism of action of, 157, 164
  side effects of, 8, 164
Chlorazepate, to treat seizures, 44, 54
Chlordane, poisoning by, 183
Chlorine, poisoning by, 184
Chloromycetin, 163
Chloroprocaine, anesthetic effect of, 77
Chloroquine
  indications for, 166
  to treat malaria, 168t
Chlorothiazide, 95, 96
  site of action of, 97t

Chlorpromazine
  antiemetic effects of, 138
  effects of, 47–49
  pharmacokinetics of, 47
  side effects of, 49–50, 51f, 52
Chlorthalidone, 95
Choleragen, 151
Cholesterol, 108
Cholestyramine
  anticholesterol effects of, 108
  to treat diarrhea, 140
Choline, 17
  receptor agonists, 18–19
Cholinergic receptors, 17–18
Cholinesterase inhibitors, 19–21
  toxicity of, 183
Choloxin, anticholesterol effects of, 108
CHOP regimen, indications for, 178
Chorioretinitis, treatment of, 166
Chromomycosis, treatment of, 165
Chronic active hepatitis, treatment of, 175
Cimetidine
  histamine$_2$ receptor blocking drug, 147
  to treat ulcer, 137
Cinobac, pharmacology of, 161
Cinoxacin, pharmacology of, 161
Ciprofloxacin, pharmacology of, 161
cis-platinum, 179
Cladosporosium infection, treatment of, 165
Clarithromycin, to treat ulcer, 138
Clofibrate, anticholesterol effects of, 108
Clomiphene, 131
Clonazepam, to treat seizures, 44
Clonidine, antihypertensive effects of, 98, 100
Clonopin, to treat seizures, 44
Clostridium infection, treatment of, 164
Cloxacillin, 162
Clozapine, 148
Central nervous system
  prostaglandin effects on, 150
  steroid effects on, 120
Central nervous system pharmacology
  alcohol, 83–85
  analgesics, 71–74
  anesthetics, 74–77
  muscle relaxants, 78–82
  narcotics, 67–70
  sedatives and hypnotics, 85
Coagulation, steroid effects on, 119
Cocaine, 27
  anesthetic effect of, 77
Coccidioidal infections, treatment of, 165
Codeine, 68
  antitussive effects of, 144
  to treat diarrhea, 140
Coenzymes, drug interactions with, 10
Cogentin
  anticholinergic effects of, 50
  to treat parkinsonism, 36
Colchicine, indications for, 73
Coliform bacteria infection, treatment of, 163
Colistin, mechanism of action of, 157
Colon cancer, treatment of, 178
COMA regimen, indications for, 178
Compactin, anticholesterol effects of, 108
Competitive antagonism, defined, 6
Congestive heart failure, treatment of, 89–91
Constipation, treatment of, 139–140
Contraceptives, 132

Copper, deficiency of, 106
Corrosives, poisoning by, 184
Corticosteroids
    classification of, 116–117
    contraindications to use of, 120
    immunosuppressive effects of, 174
    indications for, 73, 117–120, 119f
    mechanism of action of, 117–120, 121f
    pharmacology of, 175–176
    side effects of, 120f, 143
    to treat asthma, 142–143
    to treat diarrhea, 140
Corticosterone, 116
Corticotropin
    indications for, 73
    release of, 149
Cortisol, 116
Cortisone, affecting calcium levels, 128f
Coumadin, 103
Coumarin, 103
    pharmacology of, 103t
Craniosacral nervous system, 17
Creosote, expectorant effects of, 144
Cromolyn sodium, to treat asthma, 141
Cryptococcus neoformans infection, treatment of,
    165
Crystalline insulin, 113
Cuprimine, to treat poisoning, 184
CVP regimen, indications for, 178
Cyanide, poisoning by, 185
Cyclic nucleotides, synthesis of, 152
Cycloguanil embonate, indications for, 166
Cyclooxygenase, 150
Cyclophosphamide, 176
    immunosuppressive effects of, 174, 175
    indications for, 178, 179
    pharmacology of, 177
Cyclosporin A
    cytotoxic effects of, 176
    immunosuppressive effects of, 174
Cyclosporins
    drug interactions of, 154
    mechanism of action of, 157
    side effects of, 38
Cyproheptadine, 148
Cyproterone, 133
Cytarabine, 178
    indications for, 11, 178, 179
Cytochrome P-450, 7f, 8
Cytomel, 125
Cytomine, 125
Cytosine arabinoside, pharmacology of, 178
Cytostat, 178
Cytotoxic compounds, 176
    nonspecificity of, 176
Cytoxan, 176, 177

Dactinomycin, 178, 179
Dalmane, sedative effects of, 85
Dantrium, muscle relaxant effects of, 79
Dantrolene
    muscle relaxant effects of, 79
    to treat neuroleptic malignant syndrome, 52
Dapsone, indications for, 166
Daraprim, to treat malaria, 168t
Daunorubicin, 179
Dazodipine, calcium-blocking effect of, 153
Deferoxamine, 12
    to treat iron poisoning, 106, 184
Degenerative joint disease, treatment of, 73

Degree of ionization, defined, 4
Dehydroemetine, indications for, 166
Dehydroemetine resinate, indications for, 166
Deoxycytidine analogues, 178
Depakene, to treat seizures, 42, 44
L-deprenyl, 27
Depression, treatment of, 53–54, 154
Dermatophyte infection, treatment of, 165
Desipramine, 56
    indications for, 57
Desmethoxyverapamil, 153
Desmopressin acetate, 130
Dexamethasone, 116
    to treat thyrotoxic crisis, 124
Dextromethorphan, 70
    antitussive effects of, 144
Dextropropoxyphene, 69
Diabetes insipidus, 130
    treatment of, 96
Diabetes mellitus
    behavioral treatment of, 112
    drug treatment of, 112–115
    types of, 111–112
Diabetic ketoacidosis, 115
Diapid, 130
Diarrhea, treatment of, 67, 140
Diazepam
    anesthetic effect of, 74
    muscle relaxant effects of, 79
    as preanesthetic, 54
    sedative effects of, 54
    to treat alcohol withdrawal, 54
    to treat poisoning, 184, 185
    to treat seizures, 44, 54
Diazinon, 20
Diazoxide, antihypertensive effects of, 98, 99
Dibenzapine derivatives. *See* Tricyclic antidepressants
Dibenzyline, 28
Dichlorphenamide, 95
    site of action of, 97t
Dicloxacillin, 162
Dicumarol, 103
Dieldrin, poisoning by, 183
Diethyldithiocarbamate, 26
Diffuse histiocytic lymphoma, treatment of, 178
Diffusion, passive, 3
Digibind, 90
Digitalis, to treat thyrotoxic crisis, 124
Digitoxin
    drug interactions of, 154
    modes of action of, 89
    pharmacokinetics of, 89t
    side effects of, 8, 9, 90
Digoxin
    antiarrhythmic effects of, 93t
    modes of action of, 89
    pharmacokinetics of, 89t
    side effects of, 9, 90
Dihydrocodeinone, antitussive effects of, 144
Dihydrocyclosporin C, immunosuppressive effects of,
    174
Dihydropyridines, calcium-blocking effect of, 153
Diiodotyrosine (DIT), 122
Diisopropylfluorophosphate, 20, 21
Diloxanide furoate, indications for, 166
Diltiazem
    antiarrhythmic effects of, 92, 93t, 94
    antihypertensive effects of, 98, 100
    calcium-blocking effect of, 153
    cardiovascular effects of, 154t

Diltiazem (*continued*)
  drug interactions of, 154
  side effects of, 38
  to treat angina, 154
  to treat hypertension, 154
Dimercaprol, to treat poisoning, 184
Dimethylphenylpiperazinium, 18
Dinoprostone, 150
Dioctyl sodium sulfosuccinate, laxative effects of, 139
Dipaxin, 103
Diphenadione, 103
Diphenhydramine
  histamine₁ receptor blocking drug, 147
  drug interactions of, 12
  to treat dystonia, 50
Diphenoxylate, to treat diarrhea, 140
Dipropionate, to treat asthma, 143
Dipyridamole, 101
Diquat, poisoning by, 183
Disopyramide, antiarrhythmic effects of, 92, 93t, 94t
Disulfiram, 183
Diethylstilbestrol, 131
Diuretics
  affecting calcium levels, 127, 128f
  antihypertensive effects of, 98
  loop, 96
  pharmacology of, 95–96
  potassium-sparing, 96–97
  thiazide, 96
  to treat thyrotoxic crisis, 124
Diuril, 96
Dobutamine
  adrenergic activity of, 27t
  to treat congestive heart failure, 91
Docusate, laxative effects of, 139–140
Dopamine
  actions of, 32–33
  adrenergic activity of, 27t
  interaction with receptors, 48f, 50f
  metabolism of, 25
  and schizophrenia, 47
  synthesis of, 31
Dopamine blockers, as antiemetics, 138
Dose-response relationship, 6–7
Doxepin, 56
Doxorubicin, 179
Droncit, 167t
Droperidol, anesthetic effect of, 74
Drugs
  absorption of, 3–5
  administration of, 3
  adverse reactions of, 12
  bioavailability of, 3
  biotransformation of, 7–9
  distribution of, 5
  excretion of, 9
  half-life of, 9
  interactions of, 12–14
  metabolism of, 8–9
  pharmacodynamics of, 10–11
  plasma binding of, 5
  site of action of, 6
  tissue localization of, 5
  transport of, 3–4
Dyphylline, to treat asthma, 141
Dyrenium, 96
Dysentery, treatment of, 166
Dyskinesia, from levodopa, 34
Dysmenorrhea, treatment of, 71, 132, 150
Dystonia, 49–50

Ebastine, histamine₁ receptor blocking drug, 147
Echothiophate, 20
Edecrin, 96
Edema, treatment of, 96
Edetate, calcium disodium, to treat lead poisoning, 184
Edrophonium, 20, 21
Efficacy, defined, 6
Eicosanoids, 149–150
  indications for, 150
Elavil, 56
Elderly, drug metabolism in, 8
Embryonal rhabdomyosarcoma, treatment of, 179
Emesis, 139f
Emopamil, calcium-blocking effect of, 153
Enalapril, antihypertensive effects of, 98
Encainide, antiarrhythmic effects of, 92, 93, 93t
Encephalitis, treatment of, 171
Endocrine system, prostaglandin effects on, 149
Endocytosis, receptor-mediated, 4
Endometrial cancer, contraceptives and, 132
Endometriosis, treatment of, 132
Endoxan, 177
Enflurane
  anesthetic effect of, 74
  drug interactions of, 154
Enoxacin, pharmacology of, 161
Enoximone, to treat congestive heart failure, 91
Enprofylline, to treat asthma, 141
Enterobiasis, treatment of, 167t
Enuresis, treatment of, 54, 57, 59f
Enzymes, drug interactions with, 8–9
Ephedrine, as sympathomimetic, 28
Epidermophyton infection, treatment of, 165
Epilepsy
  mechanisms of, 37
  treatment of, 37–44, 54, 154
Epinephrine, 25
  adrenergic activity of, 27t
  local anesthetic effect of, 77
  to treat asthma, 141
  uses of, 27–28
Epinephrine reversal, 28
Epsilon-aminocaproic acid, 105
Erythrocin, 163
Erythromycin, mechanism of action of, 157, 163
Erythropoietin, 106
Escherichia coli infection, treatment of, 163
Eserine sulfate, 20
Esmolol
  antiadrenergic activity of, 27t, 28t
  antiarrhythmic effects of, 92, 93, 93t
Essential hypertension, treatment of, 96
Estradiol, 117
Estrogens, 131
  antagonists of, 131–132
  pharmacologic effects of, 131
Ethacrynic acid, 95, 96
  site of action of, 97t
Ethambutol, 10
  to treat tuberculosis, 168t
Ethanol
  cardiovascular effects of, 84
  central nervous system effects of, 83–84
  counteracting toxic effects of other alcohols and glycols, 183
  GI effects of, 84
  liver effects of, 85
  pharmacokinetics of, 85
  toxicity of, 183
Ether, anesthetic effect of, 74
Ethopropazine, 47

Ethosuxamide, to treat seizures, 42
Ethoxzolamide, site of action of, 97t
Ethylene glycol, poisoning by, 183
Etinidine, histamine$_1$ receptor blocking drug, 147
Etiocaine, anesthetic effect of, 77
Etomidate, anesthetic effect of, 74
Eucalyptus oil, expectorant effects of, 144
Eunuchoidism, androgens to treat, 132
Euthyroid, 125
Ewing's sarcoma, treatment of, 179
Expectorants, 144

Facilitated transport, 3
Falipamil, calcium-blocking effect of, 153
Famotidine
    histamine$_2$ receptor blocking drug, 147
    to treat ulcer, 137
Felodipine, calcium-blocking effect of, 153
Fenoldopam, 95
    to treat congestive heart failure, 91
Fenoprofen, indications for, 73
Fenoterol, to treat asthma, 141
Ferritin, 106
Fetal trimethadione syndrome, 42
Fever, prostaglandins and, 150
Flagyl, indications for, 166
Flecainide, antiarrhythmic effects of, 92, 93, 93t
Fleroxacin, pharmacology of, 161
Flordipine, calcium-blocking effect of, 153
Floxuridine, 178
Flucytosine
    drug interactions of, 165
    pharmacology of, 165
Fluid volume regulation, 96t
Flunarizine, 148
    to treat cerebrovascular disorders, 154
Flunisolide, to treat asthma, 143
Flunitrazepam, sedative effects of, 54
Fluorodeoxyuridine, 178
5-Fluorouracil, indications for, 178
Fluoxetine, 56f, 159
    indications for, 57
Fluphenazine decanoate, 47
Fluphenazine enanthate, 47
Flurazepam, sedative effects of, 85
Fluvastatin, anticholesterol effects of, 108
Folic acid
    antagonists of, 177–178
    deficiency of, 107
Follicle-stimulating hormone (FSH), 129, 152
Formoterol, to treat asthma, 141
Forskolin, 152
Fosamax, to treat osteoporosis, 127
Fruit, laxative effects of, 139
Fulvicin, 165
Fungal infection, treatment of, 165
Fungizone, 165
    indications for, 166
Furadantin, 162
Furosemide, 95, 96
    site of action of, 97t
    to treat poisoning, 183

G-protein-coupled receptors, 151
Gallopamil, calcium-blocking effect of, 153
Gamma-aminobutyric acid (GABA), 37, 38f
Ganciclovir, antiviral effects of, 171
Gas gangrene, treatment of, 163
Gastrectomy, B$_{12}$ deficiency from, 107
Gastric acid, secretion of, 147

Gastric adenocarcinoma, treatment of, 178
Gastric atony, treatment of, 19
Gastric emptying time, 5, 13
Gastrointestinal pharmacology, 137–140
Gastrointestinal smooth muscles, prostaglandin effects on, 149
General anesthetics, 74–75
Gestational choriocarcinoma, treatment of, 179
Gingival hyperplasia, 38
Glaucoma, treatment of, 19, 21, 28
Glipizide, 114
Glucagon, 111, 152
Glucocorticoids, 116
    agonists of, 116
    contraindications to use of, 120
    immunosuppressive effects of, 174
    indications for, 117–120, 119f
    mechanism of action of, 117–120, 121f
    side effects of, 120f
    to treat hyperthyroidism, 123
    to treat myxedema coma, 125
Gluconeogenesis, 111
Glucose metabolism, regulation of, 118
Glyburide, 114
Glycogen metabolism, regulation of, 118
Glycogenolysis, 111
Goitrogenic vegetables, 123
Gold sodium thiomalate, indications for, 73
Gonadotropin-releasing hormone (GnRH), 129
Gonadotropins, 152
Gonococcal infection, treatment of, 163
Gonorrhea, treatment of, 164
Gossypol, 133
Gout, treatment of, 10, 73
Gram-negative infection, treatment of, 162, 164
Gram-positive infection, treatment of, 162, 164
Granisetron, 139, 148
Granuloma inguinale, treatment of, 164
Gray baby syndrome, 8, 164
Grisactin, 165
Griseofulvin, 165
Growth hormone, 111
    deficiency of, 129
    release of, 149
Growth hormone-releasing hormone (GHRH), 129
Guanethidine
    antihypertensive effects of, 98, 99
    to treat thyrotoxic crisis, 124
Guiacols, expectorant effects of, 144

H$^+$K$^+$ ATPase inhibitors, to treat ulcer, 137–138
Haemophilus influenzae infection, treatment of, 163
Halcion, sedative effects of, 85
Half-life, drug, 9
Halogenated hydrocarbons, poisoning by, 184
Haloperidol, neuroleptic anesthetic, effect of, 74
Halothane
    anesthetic effect of, 74
    drug interactions of, 154
Head and neck cancers, treatment of, 179
Headache, treatment of, 148
Heart, stimulants for, 28
Heart disease, treatment of, 71, 89–91
Heavy metals, poisoning by, 184
Hedulin, 103
Height, estrogens to regulate, 131
Helicobacter pylori, and ulcer, 138
Hematinics, 106–107
Hemicholinium, 17
Hemiplegia, calcium channel blockers to treat, 154
Hemolysis, treatment of, 175

Heparin, 103, 105
  effects on bone, 127
  pharmacology of, 103t
Hepatic first-pass effect, 5
Hepatitis
  amoebic, treatment of, 166
  chronic, treatment of, 175
Hepatocellular carcinoma, treatment of, 178
Heptachlor, poisoning by, 183
Herbicides, poisoning by, 183
Herpes simplex infection, treatment of, 171
Herplex, 171
Hexamethonium, 18
Histamine, 138f
  actions of, 147
  receptors for, 147
Histamine$_2$ receptor blocking drug to treat ulcer, 137
HIV infection, treatment of, 171
Hodgkin's disease, treatment of, 178
Hookworm infection, treatment of, 167t
Horton's syndrome, treatment of, 148
Human immunodeficiency virus infection, treatment of, 171
Hydantoin, derivatives of, 37
Hydralazine
  antihypertensive effects of, 98, 99
  to treat congestive heart failure, 91
Hydrochloric acid
  poisoning by, 184
  steroid effects on, 119
Hydrochlorothiazide, 95, 96
  site of action of, 97t
Hydrocortisone, to treat poisoning, 183
Hydrodiuril, 96
Hydroxychloroquine, indications for, 73
Hydroxyurea, to treat cancer, 11
Hypercalcemia, 128f
Hypercalciuria, treatment of, 96
Hyperglycemia, reversal of, 115
Hyperlipoproteinemia, treatment of, 108
Hypermotility, treatment of, 148
Hyperparathyroidism, 126t, 127
Hyperstat, 99
Hypertension, treatment of, 27, 28, 154
Hypertensive crisis, treatment of, 99
Hyperthyroidism, treatment of, 122–124
Hyperuricemia, treatment of, 73
Hypnotics, 85
Hypoglycemia, 111
  from insulin therapy, 113
Hypoglycemic agents
  insulin, 112–113
  oral, 114–115
Hypogonadism, 129
  treatment of, 131, 132
Hypokalemia
  reversal of, 115
  treatment of, 96
Hypoparathyroidism, 126t, 127
Hypopituitarism, treatment of, 131, 132
Hypotension, treatment of, 28
Hypothalamic amenorrhea, 129
Hypothyroidism, treatment of, 124, 124–125
Hypoxia, calcium channel blockers to treat, 154

Iatrogenic reactions, defined, 12
Ibopamine, to treat congestive heart failure, 91
Ibuprofen, indications for, 71, 73
Idiopathic hypogonadotropic hypogonadism, 129
Idiosyncrasy, definition of, 12

Idoxuridine, antiviral effects of, 171
Ilotycin, 163
Imidazole derivatives, anesthetic effect of, 74
Iminostilbene derivatives, to treat epilepsy, 40–41
Imipramine, 24, 27, 56
  indications for, 56–57, 58f
  side effects of, 57f
Immune response, prostaglandins and, 150
Immune system, steroid effects on, 119
Immunopharmacology, 173–176
Immunosuppressants, 174–176
  indications for, 73
  sites of action of, 175f
Inanedione derivatives, 103
Indapamide, 95
Indecainide, antiarrhythmic effects of, 92, 93t
Indomethacin
  effect on ductus arteriosus, 150
  indications for, 73
Infants, drug metabolism in, 8
Inflammation
  prostaglandins and, 150
  steroid effects on, 119
Influenza A infection, treatment of, 171
Inhalational anesthetics, 74
Inhibin, synthesis of, 129
Inorganic salts, laxative effects of, 139
Inositol 1,4,5-triphosphate, calcium-facilitating effect of, 153
Insecticides, poisoning by, 183
Insulin, 152
  and diabetes, 111–112
  functions of, 111, 111f
  preparations of, 112–113
  receptor for, 112
  release of, 113–114
  side effects of, 113
Insulin edema, 113
Insulin resistance, 113
Interferons, immunosuppressive effects of, 174
Interleukin–2, 174
Intrinsic factor, defined, 3
Iodide organification, 122
Iodide trapping, 122
Iodides
  to treat hyperthyroidism, 122, 123
  to treat thyrotoxic crisis, 124
Iodine–131, 174
  to treat hyperthyroidism, 122
  to treat thyrotoxicosis, 124
Iodipine, calcium-blocking effect of, 153
Iodoquinol, indications for, 166
Ionomycin, calcium-facilitating effect of, 153
Iopanoic acid, to treat hyperthyroidism, 123
Ipecac, emetic effects of, 144
Ipodate sodium, to treat hyperthyroidism, 123
Ipratropium bromide, to treat asthma, 141, 152
Iron
  metabolism of, 106
  toxicity of, 12, 106
Irritant agents, laxative effects of, 139
Ismelin, 99
Isoflurane, anesthetic effect of, 74
Isoniazid, 10
  to treat tuberculosis, 168t
Isopropyl alcohol, poisoning by, 184
Isoproterenol
  adrenergic activity of, 27, 27t
  drug interactions of, 6–7
Isradipine, calcium-blocking effect of, 153

Kallidin, 148
Ketamine, anesthetic effect of, 74
Ketanserine, 148
Ketoacidosis, treatment of, 115
Ketoconazole, 165
Kidneys
    drug excretion from, 9
    prostaglandin effects on, 149
Kinin receptors, 148
Klebsiella pneumoniae infection, treatment of, 162, 163

Labetalol, antiadrenergic activity of, 27t, 28t
Lactation, regulation of, 131, 132
Lampit, 166
Laryngotracheitis, treatment of, 163
Lasix, 96
Laxatives, 139–140
Lead, poisoning by, 184
Leishmaniasis, treatment of, 166
Lemon oil, expectorant effects of, 144
Leprosy, treatment of, 166
Lesch-Nyhan syndrome, 10
Leucovorin, 178
Leukemia, treatment of, 178–179
Leukeran, 177
Leukocytes, steroid effects on, 119
Levocabastine, histamine$_1$ receptor blocking drug, 147
Levodopa, 25
    metabolism of, 35
    side effects of, 34
    to treat neuroleptic malignant syndrome, 52
    to treat parkinsonism, 32–35
Levorphanol, antitussive effects of, 144
Levothyroxine
    to treat hypothyroidism, 124
    to treat myxedema coma, 125
LH-releasing hormone. *See* Gonadotropin-releasing hormone
Lidocaine
    anesthetic effect of, 77
    antiarrhythmic effects of, 92, 93t, 94t
    to treat digitalis toxicity, 90
Ligand movement, 4
Linoleic acid, 149
Lioresal, muscle relaxant effects of, 79
Liothyronine, 125
Liotrix, 125
Lipid metabolism, regulation of, 118
Lipid-water partition coefficient, 4
Lipodystrophy, 113
Liquamar, 103
Lisinopril
    antihypertensive effects of, 98
    to treat congestive heart failure, 91
Lithium
    drug interactions of, 154
    excretion of, 61, 62f
    indications for, 59
    side effects of, 61–62, 63f
Liver, drug metabolism in, 8
Liver cancer
    contraceptives and, 132
    treatment of, 178
Local anesthetics, 76–77
    in treatment of diarrhea, 140
Lomotil, to treat diarrhea, 140
Lomustine, 177
Loniten, 99
Loop diuretics, 96
    effects on bone, 127

Loperamide, to treat diarrhea, 140
Loratadine, histamine$_1$ receptor blocking drug, 147
Lorazepam, 53
    anesthetic effect of, 74
Lorelco, anticholesterol effects of, 108
Losec, to treat ulcer, 137–138
Lovastatin, anticholesterol effects of, 108
Lubricants, laxative effects of, 139
Lugol's solution, to treat hyperthyroidism, 123
Luteinizing hormone (LH), 129, 152
    release of, 150
Lymphogranuloma venereum, treatment of, 164
Lymphoid irradiation, immunosuppressive effects of, 174
Lymphoma, treatment of, 179
Lypressin, 130

Magnesium citrate, laxative effects of, 139
Magnesium sulfate, laxative effects of, 139
Malabsorption syndrome, B$_{12}$ deficiency from, 107
Malaria, treatment of, 166, 168t
Malathion, 20
    poisoning by, 183
Malignant hypertension, treatment of, 99
Mandelamine, pharmacology of, 161
Mania, treatment of, 59–62, 154
Mannitol
    as diuretic, 95
    site of action of, 97t
    to treat cerebral edema, 185
MAO (monoamine oxidase) inhibitors, 58–59, 60f
Maprotiline, 58
Maxipen, 162
Mebadin, indications for, 166
Mebendazole, 167t
Mechanism of action, defined, 10
Mechlorethamine, 176
    indications for, 178
Mefenamic acid, indications for, 71
Megaloblastic anemia, 106
Melanocyte-stimulating hormone, 152
Melarsoprol, indications for, 166
Meningitis, treatment of, 163, 165
Meningococcal infection, treatment of, 163
Menopause, estrogens to treat, 131
Meperidine, 68
Mephentermine, 28
Mephenytoin, 38–39
Mephobarbital, to treat epilepsy, 40, 41f, 42f
Mepivacaine, anesthetic effect of, 77
6-mercaptopurine, 11, 176, 178
Mercury, poisoning by, 184
Mesudipine, calcium-blocking effect of, 153
Metals, poisoning by, 184
Metamucil, laxative effects of, 139
Metaproterenol, to treat asthma, 141
Methacholine, 18
Methadone, 68–69
    antitussive effects of, 144
Methanol, toxicity of, 85, 183
Methantheline, 24
Methazolamide, 95
Methenamine, pharmacology of, 161
Methicillin, 162
    side effects of, 163
Methimazole, to treat hyperthyroidism, 122, 123
Methohexital
    anesthetic effect of, 74
    sedative effects of, 85

Methotrexate, 177–178
    indications for, 178, 179
    side effects of, 160
Methoxyflurane, anesthetic effect of, 74
Methsuximide, to treat seizures, 42
Methyl-CCNU, 177
Methyl Viologen, poisoning by, 183
Methylcellulose, laxative effects of, 139
Methylprednisolone, to treat asthma, 143
Methylxanthines, to treat asthma, 141
Methysergide, 148
Metolazone, 95
Metoprolol
    antiadrenergic activity of, 27t, 28t
    antiarrhythmic effects of, 93–94
    antihypertensive effects of, 98
Metrifonate, 167t
Metronidazole, indications for, 166
Mexiletine, antiarrhythmic effects of, 92, 93, 93t
Mianserin, 59
Microsporum infection, treatment of, 165
Midamor, 96
Midazolam, anesthetic effect of, 74
Migraine
    prevention of, 154
    treatment of, 148
Milk of magnesia, laxative effects of, 139
Millontin, to treat seizures, 42
Milrinone, to treat congestive heart failure, 91
Mineralocorticoids, 116, 117
Minipress, 28, 99
Minocycline, 165
Minoxidil, 98, 99
Mintezol, 167t
Miostat, 18
Miradon, 103
Mithramycin, 179
Mixed-function oxidases, 8
Mode of action, defined, 10
Monilia infection, treatment of, 165
Monoamine oxidase, 27
    inhibitors of, 58–59, 60f
Monocytic leukemia, treatment of, 178
Monoiodotyrosine (MIT), 122
Monooxygenase, 8
MOPP regimen, 176
    indications for, 178
Moricizine, antiarrhythmic effects of, 92, 93t
Morphine, 10
    antitussive effects of, 144
    blood-brain barrier and, 6
    effects of, 67–68
    indications for, 67, 69f
    tolerance to, 12
Mucokinetics, 144
Mucolytics, 144
Mucomyst, mucolytic effects of, 144
Multiple sclerosis, 173
    treatment of, 54
Murine typhus, treatment of, 164
Muscarine, 17
Muscle relaxants, 78–82
Mustargen, 176
Muzolimine, 95
Myasthenia gravis, diagnosis of, 21
Mycobacterial diseases, treatment of, 166
Mycoplasma infection, treatment of, 164
Mycostatin, 165
Myelomonocytic leukemia, treatment of, 178
Myocardial infarction, 101

anticoagulant therapy for, 105
    aspirin in treatment of, 71
    calcium channel blockers to treat, 154
Myocardial ischemia, 101

Nadolol, antiadrenergic activity of, 27t, 28t
Nafcillin, 162
    side effects of, 163
Nalidixic acid
    mechanism of action of, 157
    pharmacology of, 161
Naloxone, 70
Naltrexone, 70
Naphthyl-*N*-methyl carbamate, poisoning by, 183
Naphuride, indications for, 166
Naproxen, indications for, 71, 73
Narcan, 70
Narcotics, 67–70
    antitussive effects of, 144
    blood-brain barrier and, 6
Nausea, treatment of, 138–139
Nedocromil sodium, to treat asthma, 141
NegGram, pharmacology of, 161
Neostigmine, 20, 21
Nervous system, divisions of, 17
Neuroleptic malignant syndrome, 52
Neuroleptics, 47–52
    anesthetic effect of, 74
    to treat diarrhea, 140
Neuromuscular blocking agents
    drug interactions of, 79–80
    factors affecting, 80
    indications for, 78f
    mechanism of action of, 79
    side effects of, 81
    types of, 79
Neuromuscular disorders, treatment of, 54
Neuropharmacology, 11, 29–44
Neurotransmitters, secretion of, 153
Niacin, deficiency of, 106
Nicardipine
    antihypertensive effects of, 98, 100, 100t
    calcium-blocking effect of, 153
Niclosamide, 167t
Nicotine, 18
Nicotinic acid, anticholesterol effects of, 108
Nifedipine
    antihypertensive effects of, 98, 100, 100t
    calcium-blocking effect of, 153
    cardiovascular effects of, 154t
    side effects of, 38
    to treat angina, 154
    to treat hypertension, 154
Nifurtimox, indications for, 166
Niludipine, calcium-blocking effect of, 153
Nimodipine, calcium-blocking effect of, 153
Nipride, 99
Niridazole, 167t
Nisoldipine, calcium-blocking effect of, 153
Nitrates
    to treat angina, 101
    to treat congestive heart failure, 91
Nitrendipine
    calcium-blocking effect of, 153
    side effects of, 38
Nitrites
    to treat angina, 101
    to treat cyanide poisoning, 185
Nitrofurantoin, 162
Nitrogen mustard, 176–177

Nitroprusside sodium, antihypertensive effects of, 98, 99
Nitrosourea, 177
Nitrous oxide, anesthetic effect of, 74
Nizatidine
    histamine₂ receptor blocking drug, 147
    to treat ulcer, 137
Nodular lymphoma, treatment of, 178
Nolvadex, 131
Norepinephrine, 25, 26f
    adrenergic activity of, 27, 27t
Norfloxacin, pharmacology of, 161
Noroxin, pharmacology of, 161
Norpramin, 56
Nortriptyline, 56
Nucleic acids, drug interactions with, 10
Nystatin, 165
    mechanism of action of, 157

Ofloxacin, pharmacology of, 161
Omeprazole, to treat ulcer, 137–138
Oncovin, 176
    indications for, 178, 179
Ondansetron, 139, 148
Opioids, 69–70
    antagonists of, 70
    to treat diarrhea, 140
Organic hydrophilic colloids, laxative effects of, 139
Organophosphorus compounds, 20, 21
    poisoning by, 183
Osteoporosis, 127
    estrogens to treat, 131
Ouabain, 27
Ovarian cancer, contraceptives and, 132
Oxacillin, 162
Oxalate, affecting calcium levels, 128f
Oxamniquine, 167t
Oxazepam, 53
    as preanesthetic, 54
Oxazolidine derivatives, to treat seizures, 42
Oxodipine, calcium-blocking effect of, 153
Oxycarbazepine, to treat epilepsy, 40–41
Oxyphenonium, 24
Oxytocin, functions of, 129

Pain
    prostaglandins and, 150
    narcotic treatments for, 67–70
    nonnarcotic treatments for, 71–74
Pancreatic cancer, treatment of, 178
Pancuronium, muscle relaxant effects of, 80
Pantothenic acid, deficiency of, 106
Paramethadione, to treat seizures, 42
Paraquat, poisoning by, 183
Parasympathetic nervous system, 17
Parathion, 20
    poisoning by, 183
Parathyroid hormone, 126, 128f
Paregoric, 67
Parkinsonism
    calcium-channel blockers and, 154
    characteristics of, 32
    mimicked by antipsychotic drugs, 50, 52
    treatment of, 25, 31–36
Paromomycin, 166
Paronychia, treatment of, 165
Parsidol, 47
Partial agonist, 7
Passive diffusion, 3
Patent ductus arteriosus, 150
Pen Vee K, 162

Penbutolol, characteristics of, 28t
D-penicillamine, indications for, 73
    to treat poisoning, 184
Penicillin
    drug interactions of, 158
    excretion of, 9, 14
    half-life of, 9
    indications for, 163
    mechanism of action of, 157, 162
    penicillinase-resistant, 162
    side effects of, 163
    types of, 162
Pentadine, indications for, 166
Pentamidine, indications for, 166
Pentavalent antimonials, indications for, 166
Pentazocine, 69–70
Pentobarbital, sedative effects of, 85
Pentoxifylline, to treat asthma, 141
Pepcid, to treat ulcer, 137
Perchlorate, to treat hyperthyroidism, 123
Perfloxacin, pharmacology of, 161
Pergolide, 33
Peripheral nervous system, 17
Pernicious anemia, 106
Perphenazine, antiemetic effects of, 138
Persantine, 101
Pertechnetate, to treat hyperthyroidism, 123
Pertussis toxin, 151–152
Petit mal, treatment of, 42–44
Petroleum products, poisoning by, 184
Pharmacodynamics, 10–11
Pharmacogenetics, 8
Phenazopyridine, 162
Phencyclidine intoxication, calcium channel blockers to treat, 154
Phenergan, 47
Phenethicillin, 162
Phenindione, 103
Phenobarbital
    drug interactions of, 13
    excretion of, 9
    sedative effects of, 85
    to treat epilepsy, 39–40, 43f
Phenol derivatives, anesthetic effect of, 74
Phenolphthalein, laxative effects of, 139
Phenothiazine derivatives, 47–52
    to treat diarrhea, 140
Phenoxybenzamine, 28
    antiadrenergic activity of, 27t
Phenprocouman, 103
Phensuxamide, to treat seizures, 42
Phentolamine, 28
    antiadrenergic activity of, 27t
Phenylalkylamines, calcium-blocking effect of, 153
Phenylbutazone
    drug interactions of, 13
    indications for, 73
Phenylethanolamine-N-methyltransferase (PNMT), 26
Phenytoin
    antiarrhythmic effects of, 92, 93t, 94t
    drug interactions of, 13
    effects on bone, 127
    to treat digitalis toxicity, 90
    to treat epilepsy, 37–38, 39f, 40f, 41f, 43f
Pheochromocytoma, treatment of, 28
Phobia, treatment of, 57
Phosgene, poisoning by, 184
Phosphate
    affecting calcium levels, 128f
    serum levels of, 126t

Physostigmine, 20, 23
  to treat tricyclic overdose, 58
Phytate, affecting calcium levels, 128f
Pilocarpine, 19
Pindolol, characteristics of, 28t
Pine oil, expectorant effects of, 144
Pinocytosis, 4
Pinworm infection, treatment of, 167t
Piperacillin, 162
Piperazine citrate, 167t
Pirenzepine, 24
  to treat ulcer, 137
Pitocin, 129
Pitressin, 130
Pituitary hormones, functions of, 129–130, 130f
Placental barrier, 5–6
Plantago seed, laxative effects of, 139
Plasma proteins, drug binding by, 5, 14
Platelets, prostaglandin effects on, 149
Pneumococcus infection, treatment of, 163
Pneumonia, treatment of, 163
Poisoning, treatment of, 183–185
Polycyclic chlorinated insecticides, poisoning by, 183
Polymyxin
  drug interactions of, 158
  mechanism of action of, 157
Postgastrectomy dumping syndrome, treatment of, 148
Potassium citrate, expectorant effects of, 144
Potassium iodide, expectorant effects of, 144
Potassium-sparing diuretics, 96–97
Potency, defined, 6
Povan, 167t
Poxvirus infection, treatment of, 171
Pralidoxime, 20
  to treat poisoning, 183
Pravastatin, anticholesterol effects of, 108
Prazepam, 53
Praziquantel, 167t
Prazosin, 28
  antiadrenergic activity of, 27t
  antihypertensive effects of, 98, 99
  drug interactions of, 154
Prednisolone, 116
  to treat asthma, 143
Prednisone
  in MOPP regimen, 176
  indications for, 178, 179
  to treat asthma, 142, 143
  to treat cerebral edema, 185
Premenstrual syndrome (PMS), treatment of, 71, 154
Prilocaine, anesthetic effect of, 77
Primaquine, to treat malaria, 168t
Primidone, to treat epilepsy, 40
Probenecid
  drug interactions of, 9, 14, 163
  indications for, 73
Probucol, anticholesterol effects of, 108
Procainamide, antiarrhythmic effects of, 92, 93t, 94t
Procaine, anesthetic effect of, 77
Procarbazine, 176
  indications for, 178
Prochlorperazine, antiemetic effects of, 138
Progesterone, 117, 131–132
  regulation of, 150
Progestins, 131–132
  side effects of, 132
Prolactin, release of, 150
Proloid, 124
Promethazine, 47
  antiemetic effects of, 138

Propafenone, antiarrhythmic effects of, 92, 93, 93t
Propamidine, indications for, 166
Propantheline, 24
  to treat ulcer, 137
Propofol, anesthetic effect of, 74
Propranolol, 28
  antiadrenergic activity of, 27t, 34
  antianginal effects of, 102
  antihypertensive effects of, 98
  antiarrhythmic effects of, 92, 93, 93t, 94t
  bronchoconstriction by, 152
  drug interactions of, 6–7
  endocrine effects of, 11
  to treat digitalis toxicity, 90
  to treat hyperthyroidism, 123
  to treat thyrotoxic crisis, 124
Propylpentanoic acid derivatives, 42, 44
Propylthiouracil
  to treat hyperthyroidism, 122, 123
  to treat thyrotoxic crisis, 124
Prostacyclin, 150
Prostaglandins, 149–150
Prostate, hypertrophy of, 133
Prostatitis, treatment of, 161
Protein kinase A, 151
Protein metabolism, regulation of, 118
Proteus infection, treatment of, 161, 163
Proton pump inhibitors, to treat ulcer, 137–138
Protozoal infections, treatment of, 166
Protriptyline, 56
Provitamin D, 127
Pseudocholinesterase deficiency, 12
Pseudomonas infection, treatment of, 163, 164
Psittacosis, treatment of, 164
Psychopharmacology
  antidepressants, 56–63
  anxiolytics, 53–55
  neuroleptics, 47–52
Psyllium, laxative effects of, 139
Pulmonary pharmacology, 141–144
Purine antimetabolites, 178
Purinergic receptors, 147
Pyrantel pamoate, 167t
Pyrazinamide, 10
Pyridium, 162
Pyridostigmine, 20, 21
Pyridoxal phosphate, 10
Pyridoxine, 10
  deficiency of, 106
Pyrimethamine
  indications for, 166
  mechanism of action of, 157
  to treat malaria, 168t
Pyrimidine analogues, 178
Pyrvinium pamoate, 167t

Q fever, treatment of, 164
Quaternary nitrogens, 20
Quelicin, muscle relaxant effects of, 79
Questran, anticholesterol effects of, 108
Quinidine, antiarrhythmic effects of, 92, 93t, 94t
Quinine, to treat malaria, 168t
Quinolones, pharmacology of, 161

Radioimmunotherapy, 174
Ranitidine
  histamine₂ receptor blocking drug, 147
  to treat ulcer, 137
Raynaud disease, treatment of, 28
Receptor, defined, 3

Receptor site, defined, 6
Receptor-mediated endocytosis, 4
Recrudescent epidemic typhus, treatment of, 164
Regitine, 28
Renal failure, treatment of, 96, 106
Renin, 11
Reproductive smooth muscles, prostaglandin effects on, 149
Reserpine, to treat thyrotoxic crisis, 124
Respiratory smooth muscles, prostaglandin effects on, 149
Restoril, sedative effects of, 85
Retrovir, antiviral effects of, 171
Reverse T_3, 122
Rhabdomyosarcoma, treatment of, 178
Rhenium-188, use in radioimmunotherapy, 174
Rheumatoid arthritis, treatment of, 73
Rhodanase deficiency, 99
RhoGAM, immunosuppressive effects of, 174
Rhubarb, laxative effects of, 139
Ribavirin, antiviral effects of, 171
Riboflavin, deficiency of, 106
Rickettsia infection, treatment of, 163, 164
Rifampin, 10
    drug interactions of, 165
    mechanism of action of, 157
    to treat tuberculosis, 168t
Rimantadine, antiviral effects of, 171
Riodipine, calcium-blocking effect of, 153
Rocky Mountain spotted fever, treatment of, 164
Romilar, 70
    antitussive effects of, 144
Ronipamil, calcium-blocking effect of, 153
Roundworm infection, treatment of, 167t
Roxatidine, histamine$_2$ receptor blocking drug, 147
Ryosidine, calcium-blocking effect of, 153

Saline laxatives, 139
Salmeterol
    adrenergic activity of, 27
    to treat asthma, 141
Salmonella infection, treatment of, 161, 163
Salt metabolism, regulation of, 117
Sarcoma, treatment of, 179
Schistosomiasis, treatment of, 167t
Schizophrenia
    symptoms of, 47
    treatment of, 47–52, 53, 154
Scopolamine, anticholinergic effects of, 22
Scrub typhus, treatment of, 164
Scurvy, 106
Secobarbital, sedative effects of, 85
Sedatives, 85
Seizures, treatment of, 37–44
Selegiline, 27
    effects on dopamine, 31, 32, 35
Semilente insulin, 113
Semustine, 177
Senna, laxative effects of, 139
Serotonin
    actions of, 148
    antagonists to, 148
    receptors for, 147–148
Serotonin blockers, as antiemetics, 138–139
Sevin, poisoning by, 183
Sex hormones, 116, 117
Shigella infection, treatment of, 161
Signal transduction, activation of, 151–152
Simbastatin, anticholesterol effects of, 108
Sintrom, 103
Site of action, defined, 10
Skeletal muscle relaxants, 78–82

Sleep disorders, treatment of, 54
Sleeping sickness, treatment of, 166
Smooth muscles, prostaglandin effects on, 149
Sodium excretion, 95
Sodium nitrite, to treat cyanide poisoning, 185
Sodium phosphate, laxative effects of, 139
Sodium sulfate, laxative effects of, 139
Solid tumors, treatment of, 179
Solvents, poisoning by, 184
Somatic nervous system, 17
Somatostatin, 129
Sotalol, antiarrhythmic effects of, 92, 93t, 94
Spare receptor, definition of, 7
Spinal anesthetics, 76, 77f
Spironolactone, 95, 96
    site of action of, 97t
Splenectomy, 175
Staphylococcus infection, treatment of, 163
Staphylococcus aureus infection, treatment of, 162
Status epilepticus, treatment of, 44
Steatorrhea, B_{12} deficiency from, 107
Steroids
    classification of, 116–117
    contraindications to use of, 120
    immunosuppressive effects of, 174
    indications for, 73, 117–120, 119f
    mechanism of action of, 117–120, 121f
    pharmacology of, 175–176
    side effects of, 120f, 143
    to treat asthma, 142–143
    to treat diarrhea, 140
Stevens-Johnson syndrome, 159
Stiff-man syndrome, treatment of, 54
Stilbamidine, indications for, 166
Stomach
    atony of, 19
    emptying time of, 5, 14
Stomach acid, secretion of, 147
Stomach cancer, treatment of, 178
Stomatitis, treatment of, 165
Stoxil, antiviral effects of, 171
Streptococcus infection, treatment of, 163
Streptokinase, 105
Streptomycin
    drug interactions of, 158
    to treat tuberculosis, 168t
Stroke, aspirin in treatment of, 71
Stuttering, calcium channel blockers to treat, 154
Succinamide derivatives, to treat seizures, 42
Succinylcholine, 12
    muscle relaxant effects of, 79, 80
    side effects of, 81
Sucostrin, muscle relaxant effects of, 79
Sulfadiazine, indications for, 166
Sulfamethoxazole, 159–161
Sulfinpyrazone, indications for, 73
Sulfonamide diuretics, site of action of, 97t
Sulfonamides
    mechanism of action of, 157
    pharmacology of, 159
    resistance to, 161f
Sulfonylureas, 114–115
Sulfoxone, indications for, 166
Sulindac, indications for, 73
Sumatriptan, 148
Supersensitivity, defined, 12
Suramin, indications for, 166
Surface area, defined, 4
Surmountable antagonism, defined, 6
Sux-Cert, muscle relaxant effects of, 79

Symmetrel, antiviral effects of, 171
Sympathetic nervous system, 17
Sympathomimetics, 28
Syncillin, 162
Syntocinon, 129
Syphilis, treatment of, 163, 164

T_3, 122
T_4, 122
   effects on calcium and phosphorus, 126t, 127
   synthesis of, 124f
Tachyarrhythmias, 92
Tachyphylaxis, 12
Taenia infection, treatment of, 167t
Tagamet, to treat ulcer, 137
Talwin, 69–70
Tamoxifen, 131
Tapeworm
   B_{12} deficiency from, 107
   treatment of, 167t
Tardive dyskinesia, 50, 52
Telenzepine, to treat ulcer, 137
Temazepam, sedative effects of, 85
Terbutaline, to treat asthma, 141
Terfenadine, histamine₁ receptor blocking drug, 147
Tertiary nitrogens, 20
Testicular cancer, treatment of, 178
Testosterone, 117, 132
   synthesis of, 129
Tetanus, treatment of, 54
Tetracaine, anesthetic effect of, 77
Tetracycline
   absorption of, 12
   indications for, 164
   mechanism of action of, 157
   side effects of, 164
Tetraethyl pyrophosphate (TEPP), poisoning by, 183
Tetraethylammonium, 18
Tetrahydrobiopterin, 25
Theophylline
   drug interactions of, 154
   to treat asthma, 141
Therapeutic index, 7
Thiabendazole, 167t
Thiazide diuretics, 96
   antihypertensive function of, 98
Thiocyanate, to treat hyperthyroidism, 123
6-thioguanine, 178
Thiopental
   anesthetic effect of, 74
   sedative effects of, 85
Thioperamide, 147
Thioridazine, 23–24
Thoracolumbar nervous system, 17
Thrombocytopenic purpura, treatment of, 175
Thrombolytics, 103, 105
Thromboxane A, 150
Thyroglobulin, 124
Thyroid cancer, treatment of, 179
Thyroid hormones
   antagonists of, 123–124
   regulation of, 122
   synthesis of, 122
Thyroid-stimulating hormone (TSH), 122, 152
Thyrolar, 125
Thyrotoxicosis, 124
Thyrotropin, 122
Thyrotropin-releasing hormone (TRH), 122, 152
Thyroxine, 122
   anticholesterol effects of, 108

effects on calcium and phosphorus, 126t, 127
   synthesis of, 124f
Thyroxine-binding globulin (TBG), 122
Thyroxine-binding prealbumin (TBPA), 122
Ticarcillin, 162
Tienilic acid, site of action of, 97t
Timolol
   antiarrhythmic effects of, 93–94
   characteristics of, 28t
Tissue transplantation, 173–174
Tocainide, antiarrhythmic effects of, 92, 93, 93t
Tofranil, 56
Tolerance, defined, 12
Tolmetin, indications for, 73
Toluene, poisoning by, 184
Torulopsis glabrata infection, treatment of, 165
Toxoplasmosis, treatment of, 166
Transferrin, 106
Transplantation, complications of, 173–174
Transport, mechanisms of, 3–4
Tranxene, to treat seizures, 44, 54
Tranylcypromine, 27, 60f
Trazodone, 59
Trexan, 70
Triamcinolone, 116
   to treat asthma, 143
Triamterene, 95, 96
   site of action of, 97t
Triazolam, sedative effects of, 85
Trichloroethylene, poisoning by, 184
Trichophyton infection, treatment of, 165
Trichuriasis, treatment of, 167t
Tricyclic antidepressants, 56–58
   indications for, 56–57
   side effects of, 56, 58
Triethylperazine, antiemetic effects of, 138
Triflupromazine, antiemetic effects of, 138
Trifluridine, antiviral effects of, 171
Trihexyphenidyl
   anticholinergic effects of, 50
   to treat parkinsonism, 36
Triiodothyronine, 122
Trimethadione, to treat seizures, 42
Trimethoprim
   combination with sulfamethoxazole, 159–161
   mechanism of action of, 157
Tromethamine, 150
Trophic hormones, 152
Tropisetron, 148
Trypanosomiasis, treatment of, 166
Tubarine, muscle relaxant effects of, 79
Tuberculosis, treatment of, 10, 166, 168t
D-tubocurarine, 18, 21
   muscle relaxant effects of, 79, 80
   side effects of, 81
Tularemia, treatment of, 164
Turpentine, expectorant effects of, 144
Typhoid fever, treatment of, 163
Typhus, treatment of, 164
Tyramine, 12
   as sympathomimetic, 28
Tyrosine hydroxylase, 25

Ulcers, treatment of, 137–138
Ultralente insulin, 113
Urea
   as diuretic, 95
   site of action of, 97t
Urecholine chloride, 18
Uric acid, steroid effects on, 119

Urinary retention, treatment of, 19
Urinary tract infection, treatment of, 160–161, 161–162, 164
Urokinase, 105
Uteracon, 129
Uterine bleeding, treatment of, 131, 132

V-Cillin K, 162
Vaginitis, treatment of, 131, 165
Valium
    muscle relaxant effects of, 79
    to treat seizures, 44, 54
Valproic acid, to treat seizures, 42, 44
Vancomycin, mechanism of action of, 157
Vanquin, 167t
Vansil, 167t
Vascular smooth muscle, prostaglandin effects on, 149
Vasodilators, antihypertensive effects of, 98, 99
Vasopressin, 95, 130, 152
Venous thrombosis, treatment of, 104
Venous vasodilators, 98, 99
Verapamil
    antiarrhythmic effects of, 92, 93t, 94
    antihypertensive effects of, 98, 100, 100t
    calcium-blocking effect of, 153
    cardiovascular effects of, 154t
    drug interactions of, 154
    side effects of, 38
    to treat angina, 154
    to treat digitalis toxicity, 90
    to treat hypertension, 154
    to treat psychiatric disorders, 154
Vermox, 167t
Vibrio cholerae, toxin produced by, 151
Vidarabine, antiviral effects of, 171
Vinblastine, 178–179
Vinca alkaloids, 178

Vincristine, 176, 178, 179
    indications for, 178–179
Vindesine, 178
Vitamin A, transport of, 4
Vitamin B_{12}
    deficiency of, 106
    transport of, 3
Vitamin C, 25
    deficiency of, 106
Vitamin D, 127
    transport of, 4
Vitamin E, transport of, 4
Vitamin K, transport of, 4
Vivactil, 56
Volatile oils, expectorant effects of, 144
Volume of distribution, defined, 5
Vomiting, treatment of, 138–139

Warfarin, 103
Water metabolism, regulation of, 117, 119
Wilms' tumor, treatment of, 179
Wilson's disease, treatment of, 175

Xanthine oxidase, inhibition of, 10
Xylene, poisoning by, 184

Yeast infection, treatment of, 165
Yomesan, 167t
Yttrium-90, use in radioimmunotherapy, 174

Zacopride, 139
Zantac, to treat ulcer, 137
Zarontin, to treat seizures, 42
Zidovudine, 106
    antiviral effects of, 171
Zinc, deficiency of, 106
Zyloprim, indications for, 73